3 Shake the child firmly by th
shout into the ear. If no respo

Large child (approx. 8 yrs, or over)

Airway 4 Roll the child onto one side. Turn the head slightly
downwards. Clear the mouth.
- Tilt the child's head back, and lift the jaw.

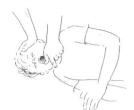

Breathing 5 Listen, look and feel for breathing. If the child is not
breathing, apply mouth-to-mouth resuscitation.
- Place the child on the back, and open the airway, as above.
- Pinch the child's nose, and place your mouth over the child's mouth.
- Give 5 full breaths in 10 seconds.
- Check pulse over 5 seconds.
- If there is no pulse, ⬇ CIRCULATION.
- If there is a pulse but no breathing, give 1 full breath every 4 seconds.

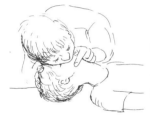

6 Keep repeating this procedure until the ambulance arrives or the child starts breathing.
7 Check the pulse after 1 minute, then every 2 minutes.
8 If the child vomits, ⬆ AIRWAY. If there is no pulse, ⬇ CIRCULATION.

Circulation 9 If there is no pulse, use CPR (cardiopulmonary resuscitation — mouth-to-mouth resuscitation and chest compressions).
- Place the heel of one hand on the lower half of the child's breastbone, and grip your wrist with the other hand.
- Press down about 4–5 cm.
- Give 15 compressions, then 2 breaths, every 15 seconds (2 people: 5 compressions, then 1 breath, every 5 seconds).

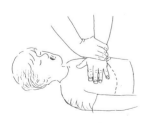

10 Keep repeating this procedure until the ambulance arrives or the pulse returns.
11 Check the pulse after 1 minute, then every 2 minutes.
12 If the pulse returns, ⬆ BREATHING.
13 If the pulse and breathing return, ⬆ AIRWAY.
14 If the child vomits during resuscitation, ⬆ AIRWAY.

See pp. 26–34 for more detail.

Jennifer Brown is a Safety Consultant at the Royal Children's Hospital, Melbourne. For many years she has conducted education programmes for parents, childcare professionals and health service providers, and community groups. Jennifer is particularly interested in health promotion and resource development.

Tony Walker is an Intensive Care Paramedic with Ambulance Service Victoria. He has a special interest in child-based first aid and resuscitation, and has developed courses for the Royal Children's Hospital Safety Centre and Emergcare. Tony frequently lectures on paediatric pre-hospital care to parents, caregivers and professional groups.

Royal Children's Hospital, Melbourne

Safety & First Aid Book

A practical guide to • emergency first aid
• safety • injuries • illnesses

Jennifer Brown & Tony Walker

Lothian
B O O K S

The Royal Children's Hospital Safety Centre has consulted widely in the development of this book. Wherever possible, the first aid and resuscitation techniques have been based on the guidelines of the Australian Resuscitation Council. This book is designed as an information text only. The authors and publisher accept no responsibility for damages caused by following the procedures in this book.

Recommended first aid procedures outlined in this text may change over time. Many of the procedures outlined, such as resuscitation, can only be learnt with a trained instructor. Information on first aid courses can be obtained from the Royal Children's Hospital Safety Centre or your local Ambulance Service. In the event of an emergency, an ambulance service or doctor should be contacted without delay.

The safety and health information is the most current information available at the time of publication, and may be subject to change. For further advice contact the Royal Children's Hospital Safety Centre. Every effort has been made to ensure that the content is accurate and reflects generally accepted safety and first aid practices. The information in this book will be reviewed constantly, and appropriate changes will be included in future editions

The Royal Children's Hospital, Melbourne, wishes to acknowledge The Pratt Foundation for their generous financial support, which made this book possible.

Thomas C. Lothian Pty Ltd
11 Munro Street, Port Melbourne, Victoria 3207

Copyright © Safety Centre, Royal Children's Hospital, Melbourne, 1996
First published 1996

National Library of Australia
Cataloguing-in-Publication data:

Brown, Jennifer, 1956- .

The Royal Children's Hospital, Melbourne, safety & first aid book.

Includes index.
ISBN 0 85091 775 1.

I. First aid in illness and injury. I. Walker, Tony, 1963- .
II. Royal Children's Hospital (Melbourne, Vic.).
III. Title.

616.0252

Produced and typeset by The Modern Art Production Group
Illustrations by Jocelyn Bell
Printed by PT Pac-Rim Kwartanusa Printing, Indonesia

Foreword

One of the truly frustrating things about young children is the variety of ways in which they can manage to injure themselves. Parents have to be one jump ahead of what they might be likely to get up to, and it is up to every one of us to make a child's environment as safe as possible.

Some of the predicaments children get into you just can't imagine! But the experts at the Royal Children's Hospital Safety Centre in Melbourne can. It is their job to find out how accidents happen and to figure out practical strategies to prevent them from happening. Their book provides sensible, achievable advice on anything from the way you set up your kitchen or the clothes you choose for your children, to the temperature you set for your hot water service.

When you are the first at the scene of a medical emergency, you will need to act quickly and decisively. Basic first aid measures are also presented in a clear, easy-to-follow way.

The staff of the Royal Children's Hospital Safety Centre, and in particular the authors Jennifer Brown and Tony Walker, are to be congratulated for sharing their valuable information in the publication of this *Safety & First Aid Book*. With the co-operation of an impressive list of reviewers, this makes a unique collaboration of experts in all areas of child health and safety. All parents and childcarers can now benefit from their combined expertise. One life saved, or one injury prevented, will have made all their efforts worthwhile.

We all worry about the wellbeing of our children. Perhaps we will all worry a little less if we know we have done whatever we can to prevent an accident, and we are prepared to handle any emergency situation with confidence.

Dr Kerryn Phelps

Dr Kerryn Phelps is a general practitioner in Sydney, and an Associate in the Department of General Practice at the Royal North Shore Hospital. She is also Australia's best-known health commentator, regularly presenting health information on TV, and in newspapers and magazines.

How to use this book

Each chapter has three sections:
- Facts
- Prevention
- First aid.

A quick page reference is given on the front flap to direct you to the **emergency first aid sections** for some of the more common injuries and illnesses.

The first few chapters of the book are essential reading. They include:
- ways to prevent accidents
- how to be prepared for injury or illness
- emergency life-support techniques.

Everyone should know first aid and resuscitation. This *Safety & First Aid Book* is not a substitute for doing a formal first aid course and learning the skills first hand, but it will take you through the necessary steps and give you the confidence to try. If you have completed a first aid course specialising in babies and children, this book will be a great reminder of what you have learnt. It's bound to include much more than you already know.

The **Life-threatening emergencies chart** (front flap) summarises the procedures to follow when caring for a child in an emergency. It is a brief guide only. You should read the complete chapter on life-threatening emergencies to gain a better understanding of how to cope with such emergencies.

Contents

Contents

Acknowledgements

Many individuals and organisations were consulted and contributed to the production of this book.

A special thanks to Lynda Hannah and Jan Shield, Safety Centre, Royal Children's Hospital, Melbourne, for their encouragement, support and expertise; to Alison Walker, Manager, Client Services, Emergcare, for her continuing support; and Jocelyn Bell, Artist, Educational Resources Centre, Royal Children's Hospital, Melbourne, for her dedication and wonderful illustrations.

We also thank the following people who reviewed and commented on chapters: Joan Adams, Road Safety Department, VicRoads; Dr Tony Catto-Smith, Department of Gastroenterology, Royal Children's Hospital, Melbourne; Dr John Court, Centre for Adolescent Health, Royal Children's Hospital, Melbourne; Diana Courtney, The Asthma Foundation of Victoria; Raylee Crutchfield, Infection Control, Royal Children's Hospital, Melbourne; Mr James Elder, Department of Ophthalmology, Royal Children's Hospital, Melbourne; Dr Hamish Farrow, Department of Plastic Surgery, Royal Children's Hospital, Melbourne; Anne Ferrie, Maternal and Child Health, Royal Children's Hospital, Melbourne; Rebecca Gebert, Department of Endocrinology and Diabetes, Royal Children's Hospital, Melbourne; Kay Gibbons, Nutrition and Food Services, Royal Children's Hospital, Melbourne; Professor Kerr Graham, Department of Orthopaedics, Royal Children's Hospital, Melbourne; Kerry Haynes, Centre for Community Child Health & Ambulatory Paediatrics, Royal Children's Hospital, Melbourne; Liz Hender, Victorian Poisons Information Centre, Royal Children's Hospital, Melbourne; Dr Sian Hughes, Consulting Paediatrician, Royal Children's Hospital, Melbourne; Mr Julian Keogh, Burns Unit, Royal Children's Hospital, Melbourne; Mr G. L. Klug, Department of Neurosurgery, Royal Children's Hospital, Melbourne; Dr Rosemary Lester, Infectious Diseases Unit, Department of Human Services Victoria; Ethna Macken, Maternal & Child Health, Royal Children's Hospital, Melbourne; Professor Frank Oberklaid, Centre for Community Child Health & Ambulatory Paediatrics, Royal Children's Hospital, Melbourne; Barry Parsons, Pharmacy, Royal Children's Hospital, Melbourne; Diana Sawyer, Epilepsy Foundation of Victoria; Sue Scott, Infection Control, Royal Children's Hospital, Melbourne; Dr Lloyd Shield, Department of Neurology, Royal Children's Hospital, Melbourne; Dr Mike South, Department of General Paediatrics, Royal Children's Hospital, Melbourne; Dr James Tibballs, Intensive Care Unit, Royal Children's Hospital, Melbourne; Dr John Williamson, Hyperbaric Medicine Unit, Royal Adelaide Hospital.

Many thanks to Michèle Adler, Department of Agriculture Forestry & Horticulture, University of Melbourne, who researched and assisted in the writing of the section on poisonous plants; and Dr John Sheahan, Department of Dentistry, Royal Children's Hospital, Melbourne, for his significant contribution to the chapters on teeth injuries and tooth decay.

Statistics were provided by the Victorian Injury Surveillance System and the National Injury Surveillance Unit.

Many thanks also to the following people who assisted throughout the production stage of this book: Jo Allan; Susan Anderson; Sharryn Bowman; Holly Brown; Nicholas Brown; Noelene Bullock; Boon Chia; Daniel Chia; Jack Dooley; Alexandra Egan; Chris Egan; Nadia Farah; Renate Ferns; Crystal Fielder; Bernie Harkins; Louise Hester; Jessica Huynh; Katra Ismile; Paul-Yung Low; Stephen McGeehan; Graham McGrath; Anna McGonigal; Jon Pogson; Jacqui Randall; Carole Regan; Marie Tan; Julie VanBavel; Andrew Walker; Teresa Williams; Ana Yoannides; and to the many parents and children who so willingly told their story.

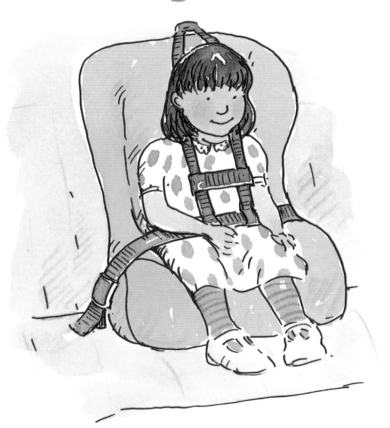

Safety

Growing up safely

The risk of injury

Childhood is a time to explore, to learn new things, make new friends, discover the world and dream the impossible! We all want the best for our children, and try to protect them from any harm. Parents feel an overwhelming sense of responsibility for the health and wellbeing of their child right from birth, and this continues throughout life. You will constantly be faced with deciding just how much freedom to allow your children to give them the opportunity to learn, against protecting them at all times.

Children, particularly young children, are at risk of injury because of their size and lack of understanding of dangers. They become overly excited, adventurous and easily distracted. As they get older, some children try to impress their friends, and take unnecessary risks. By understanding the stages of growth and knowing what to expect, you will be taking an important step towards safeguarding your child.

What follows is a brief guide to some of the stages of child development and safety hints relevant to each age. It is important to realise that not all children will go through the developmental stages at exactly the same age; some children reach a stage later or earlier than others. This is normal.

It is always a good idea to plan ahead for safety. Do not wait until your child reaches a certain stage before acting. You need to be well prepared so that you are not taken by surprise. If your child has a disability and development is delayed, always use safety strategies suited to the child's developmental age, not the actual age. Below are a few basic safety ideas, there are many more throughout the book. See also **Why accidents happen and how to prevent them** (pp. 9–19).

The growing years

The first year of life is a time of rapid growth and development for a baby. It is also a time of major change for parents as you learn to adjust to a completely different lifestyle and routine, and your new baby seems so vulnerable and dependent upon you.

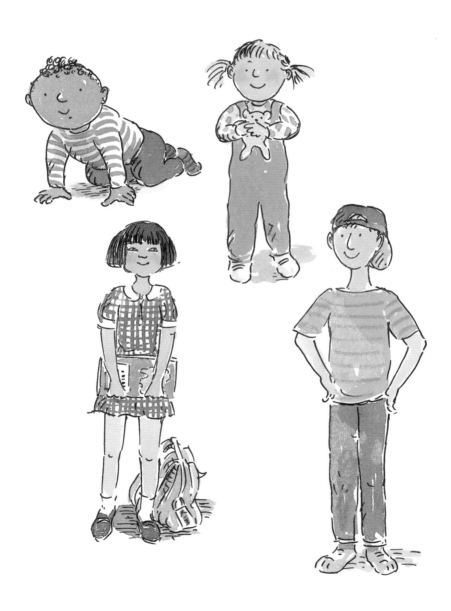

3

Birth to 3 months
- Wriggles, starts to kick and roll, raises head.
- Grasps an object when it is placed in the hand.
- Cries and smiles.
- Starts to settle into a routine of feeding and sleeping.

Safety hints
* Buy a car restraint and nursery furniture that meet Australian standards.
* Use a bassinet, or fold the blankets so that the baby sleeps at the bottom end of the cot.
* Use blankets, not a doona, and avoid cot bumpers.
* Do not leave your baby alone on a bed, table, chair or couch.
* Choose a change table with a restraining strap, and always keep one hand firmly on the baby, or change the baby on the floor.
* Avoid nursing the baby when you are having a hot drink.
* Keep the baby well away from family pets.
* Set your hot water system to 50–55°C, and fit temperature control devices or safety taps.

By 6 months
- Wriggles, kicks, rolls over.
- Grasps objects.
- Puts everything into mouth.
- Starts to sit up.
- Babbles.
- First tooth may appear (can be earlier or later).

Safety hints
* Keep small objects well out of reach.
* Use a full shoulder-harness in a high chair, pram or stroller.
* Keep your baby out of the sun, use shade, a hat and clothing.
* Remove strings or cords from clothing and toys.

By 9 months
- Sits up on own.
- Crawls.
- Can stand holding onto a hand or furniture.
- Tries to climb.
- Responds to own name.
- Says 'mama' and 'dada'.

Safety hints

* Use barriers on the top and bottom of stairs, and in the doorway of the bathroom, kitchen and laundry.
* Place a guard around the heater or fire, and attach the guard securely to the wall.
* Lock medicines and household cleaning products away.
* Make sure the nappy bucket has a tight lid, and place it out of reach.
* Supervise your baby near any water.
* Install a safety switch, and use power-point covers.
* Place plastic covers on the corners of a low table.
* Choose 'Low fire danger' nightwear.
* Keep indoor plants well out of reach.
* Adjust the harness in the child's car seat every time you use it.

Energetic and curious **toddlers** are at high risk of injury, as they have very little fear or understanding of dangers. They like to explore, try new things, and practise their skills.

By 1 year
* Pulls up to stand without help.
* Takes first steps with one hand held.
* Will move about, grabbing onto furniture.
* May speak a few words.

Safety hints
* Teach your child to sit quietly to eat.
* Keep hot drinks, kettles and saucepans out of reach.
* Use the back burners, and place a guard around the top of the stove.
* Empty the paddling pool every time after use.
* Install a fence approved by Standards Australia around a backyard pool or spa, with a self-latching, self-closing gate.
* Protect your child from the sun, using shade, a hat and clothing; apply sunscreen sparingly on hands, feet and face.

By 2 years
* Runs and jumps.
* Climbs furniture and stairs alone, one step at a time.
* Can walk backwards.
* Turns knobs, dials and taps, and unscrews lids.
* Able to feed self, and helps with putting clothes on.
* Takes off shoes and socks.
* Listens to stories, and will point to pictures and turn pages.
* Starts putting sentences together.

Safety hints
* Continue to supervise your child in the bath.
* Maintain the hot water system at 50–55°C, fit temperature control devices or safety taps.
* Fit shatter-resistant film to low glass.
* Keep matches and sharp knives locked away.
* Provide a safe, fenced, playing area away from roads or water.
* Praise your child for keeping the car seat harness on.

Preschoolers are busy people and fiercely independent. They have a poor but growing sense of their own safety, and are better able to follow directions. They can have a vivid imagination, and do not know the difference between fantasy and reality. They will tend to copy what others do, so setting them a good example is important.

By 4 years
* Starts to count.
* Tells stories, and plays pretend games.
* Copies pictures, and likes to draw, cut and paste.
* Likes more active and fast-paced games.
* May be reckless.
* Has a short attention span, and no concept of time.
* Can ride a tricycle.
* Goes to the toilet alone.

Safety hints
* Hold your child's hand near traffic.
* When bicycling in the backyard, the child should wear a bicycle helmet.
* Start swimming lessons.
* Choose low play equipment with soft undersurfacing.
* Supervise your child near pets, particularly dogs, at all times.
* Use a booster seat with a child harness (an H-harness). See **car restraint weight limits** (p. 15).

Starting school will be a big event for both parent and child, and your youngster will seem to grow up very fast. Despite being generally more aware, children of this age still need reminders about their own and others' safety. They have difficulty applying their knowledge in new situations.

By 6 years
* Curious and adventurous.
* Easily distracted.
* Can misjudge the distance and speed of cars.
* Does not reason very well to foresee the results of actions.

Safety hints

* Do not take a child's ability, knowledge or commonsense for granted, they still need lots of supervision, particularly in new situations.
* Teach children to 'Stop, Look, Listen, and Think' before and while crossing roads.
* Closely supervise your child near all traffic.
* Set the right example by using lights or a pedestrian crossing when they are available.
* When bicycling, your child should be supervised, wear a helmet, and ride on a bike path or in the backyard.

By 9 years

• Better able to understand and judge traffic.
• Generally more responsible.
• Can sometimes be silly, and get carried away with friends.

Safety hints

* Allow your child to cross quiet roads alone, but you must supervise at busy ones.
* A child is best playing a sport with modified rules.
* Reinforce the need for the child to wear a bicycle helmet.

The transition from childhood to **adolescence** can be exciting, yet confusing at times. Older children and teenagers are often risk-takers, and can be easily influenced by their friends. Their interests and energy are often channelled into sports and other recreational interests such as bicycling, rollerblading (in-line skating) or competitive sports. Sports injuries occur more often in this group, sometimes because of the lack of protective equipment, such as bicycle helmets or mouthguards.

By 12 years

• Tries to be more assertive and independent.
• More co-ordinated and physically stronger.
• Good understanding of the consequences of their behaviour.

Safety hints

* When rollerblading (in-line skating) or skateboarding, a child should wear a helmet, wrist, elbow and knee protectors.
* Supervise when the child is lighting barbecues or fires.
* Warm-up and cool-down exercises before and after sport are necessary.

By 15 years

- Experiences rapid physical and emotional changes.
- As teenagers are under pressure to be like their friends, they are easily influenced by them.
- Can be sensible one day and impulsive the next.
- Some teenagers consider safety secondary to fashion, comfort and the opinions of their friends.
- Tend to experiment and push things, including parents, to the limit.

Safety hints

* Set firm guidelines, allowing for some flexibility and maintain routines.
* Praise and encourage sensible decision-making.
* Recognise their achievements.
* Set a good example.
* Discuss safety rules and the reasons for them, including the consequences of taking risks.
* Insist on the use of a bicycle helmet, and protective equipment when playing sport.
* Make rules for attending parties, and ensure arrangements for coming home at night are satisfactory.
* Encourage a balanced approach to meals, sleep, study and exercise.

It is not easy, but by trying to keep a few steps ahead of your fast-developing child you will ensure a safe and happy childhood.

Why accidents happen, and how to prevent them

Facts

Did you know . . .
- Injury is the highest cause of death of Australian children and adolescents.
- Twice as many boys as girls are injured.
- Drowning is the greatest cause of death of children under 5 years of age.
- Pedestrian accidents are the greatest cause of death of children aged between 5 and 9 years.
- Sports and recreational injuries are highest for children 10 to 14 years of age.
- More children from low-income and non-English-speaking backgrounds are injured.

There are many ways you can protect your child from being injured. You are probably doing a lot already. You have learnt from your own experience and from others, and developed some good safe habits over the years. You use safety products, and your general knowledge about safety continues to increase. You are reading this book now.

If you are about to become a parent for the first time, you may feel excited and at the same time apprehensive about what lies ahead. There will be many new experiences and a lot to learn, and now is the best time to find out as much as you can. You will have to make many important decisions; for example, what nursery furniture or car restraint should you choose? By getting the right advice now you will be well on the way to creating a safe future for your child. Of course, once your baby arrives, expect to learn much more 'on the job'!

It may not be all that surprising to know that many accidents during the week happen between 4 p.m. and 9 p.m. in the home. Why? Because it's the end of a busy day, everyone is tired, the children are active and there's still a lot to be done before finally going to bed. When parents or children are tired, feeling stressed, or simply because there is too much going on, the chances of an accident occurring increases. Rest, relaxation, or 'taking some time out' for yourself, can make a difference.

It is simply impossible to watch your child 24 hours a day. Designing your house for safety has proved to be one of the best ways to prevent accidents.

Throughout this book we give information about preventing injuries. Some of the sections you may wish to refer to for more detailed information include:

Bites and stings
Bleeding
Bone, muscle and joint injuries
Burns
Choking, suffocation and strangulation
Drowning
Eye injuries
Head injuries
Needle-stick injuries
Poisoning
Teeth injuries
Traffic accidents

Safe houses

You can't 'child proof' your home, you can only try to make it 'child resistant'! By adding a safety product or taking dangerous objects away, you are making it harder for your child to be injured. Once you have made the change you can relax, but you can't afford to be too complacent. Some strategies are more effective than others, and some children more determined than others.

When you are renovating or building a house it gives you a perfect opportunity to include some special safety features. For example, ducted heating is safer than an open fire. Temperature-control devices and specially designed hot water systems reduce the risk of hot water burns. Non-slip flooring lowers the risk of falling. In fact, every room in the house can be designed to include some safety feature. There are many choices you can make, and some cost little or almost nothing.

Houses are often designed and built for adults, and it isn't until a new baby arrives that we discover how unsafe the houses are. Adding safety products will help. It isn't necessary to buy every safety product. Some are better than others. Some products are a must — for example, smoke detectors, and cupboard locks to store poisons and medicines. Throughout this book, you will be referred to a selection of safety products, and an explanation of each is included in this chapter. There are many more.

Look around your home, and consider what possible dangers or hazards are present from a child's perspective. Depending upon the ages of your children, select those safety products best suited to your situation. Sometimes teaching your child, or yourself, to do something safely can be just as effective. Test yourself by completing the whole home safety checklist at the end of this chapter.

Can you find all eight safety features in this illustration?

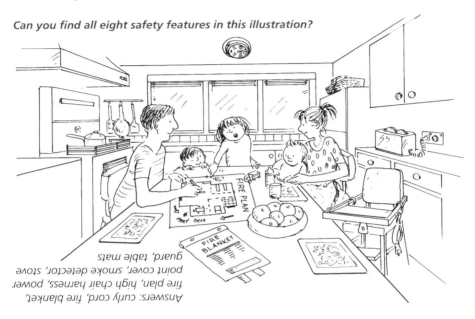

Answers: curly cord, fire blanket, fire plan, high chair harness, power point cover, smoke detector, stove guard, table mats

Outdoor safety

The backyard is an adventure playground for active and energetic children. If you plan to install play equipment, get some advice about what to look for, and how to set it up. There are Australian standards for playground equipment, and organisations such as the Playgrounds and Recreation Association of Victoria can offer specialist advice.

Young children are particularly at risk of drowning, and must be supervised closely near any water, both inside and outside the house. Outside pools and spas, whether above or below the ground, should be fenced on all sides with a fence approved by Standards Australia, and have a self-closing, self-latching gate maintained in good working order. Fish ponds, buckets of water or drains can be equally dangerous for children playing in the backyard. Cover the fishpond securely with mesh, and cover up drains or holes that fill with water after heavy rain.

The doors of the garage and garden shed should be locked, and any poison, pesticide, flammable liquid, or power tool such as an electric drill or saw,

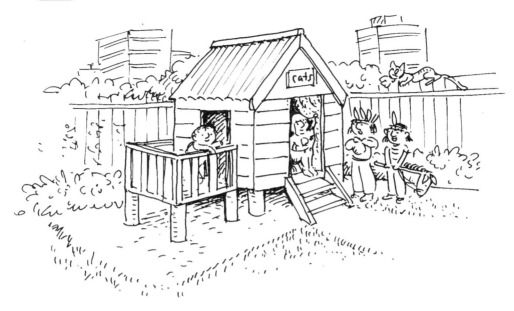

stored in locked cupboards. Make a point of cutting the grass regularly, and keeping the backyard free of rubbish. These areas sometimes provide a home for spiders, wasps, bees, mosquitoes, and even snakes. Check for poisonous plants, and remove them if necessary, see **Poisonous plants** (pp. 106–9).

Safety in the car

Australian Standard
AS 1754
Standards Australia

Child car restraints, when correctly used, have proved to be effective in preventing serious injuries to babies and children in a car crash. The restraint must fit the child's body and be correctly installed in the car. As a child's body is smaller, weighs less and is more fragile than an adult's body, an adult seat belt is not suitable. Expect to use two or three different child restraints before your child is big enough to use an adult seat belt.

By law, child restraints sold in Australia must meet certain safety standards. These child restraints display the Australian Standard AS1754 sticker. There are many different types of restraints, brands and models available.

Children with special needs, a medical condition or a physical disability may need a specially designed seat or be fitted into one of the available child restraints by an occupational therapist, a physiotherapist or a professionally trained safety consultant at your local Children's Hospital.

Be careful if you are thinking about buying a secondhand restraint. Ask the person who is selling the restraint about its background. You want to make sure that the restraint hasn't been in an accident, that it isn't over ten years old, and is still in good condition. Don't buy a restraint that is cracked, has frayed straps or a buckle that is hard to use or close. If in doubt, don't buy it! If you do decide to buy the restraint, make sure you get the instruction booklet, which tells you how to use it and install it correctly in your car.

The child restraint you need depends upon your child's weight and size. See **Child car restraints: types and maximum weight limits** (p. 15). Children of the same age differ in weight and size, and therefore there are no hard-and-fast rules about age limits. It is always best to leave a child in a seat until the child has outgrown it, rather than move to the next stage too early.

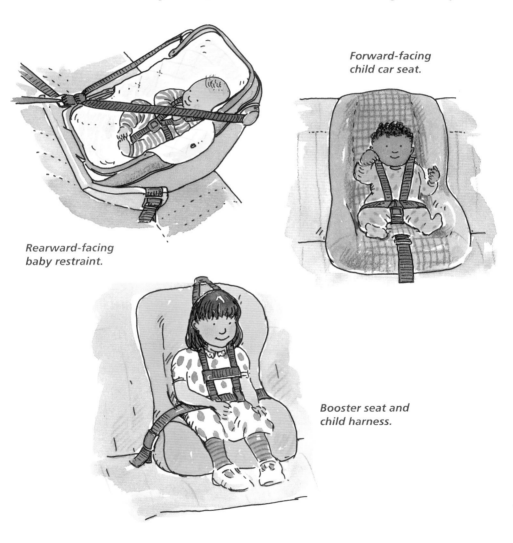

Forward-facing child car seat.

Rearward-facing baby restraint.

Booster seat and child harness.

13

The back seat is safer than the front seat; however, the lap belt in the centre back position (when used on its own) is unsuitable for children.

Child car seats for children weighing up to 18 kg must be attached to the car using a seat belt and bolt. There are two types of bolts, the old key snap-down bolt and the newer clip-on bolt. Some restraints fit better in some cars than others. Ask if you can try before you buy a seat, or, if necessary, replace it with another one. If you need advice about the range of restraints available, or how to correctly fit them, phone a child restraint fitting station, road safety authority or child safety organisation in your state or territory.

Your child will watch you closely as you do up your own seat belt, and learn to follow your example. Be consistent, and make sure that everyone in the car is restrained at all times.

Sometimes a toddler will get restless and try to get out of the child car seat. Be firm, and give plenty of encouragement and praise when the child co-operates. Try distracting your child with a soft toy, audiotape, or a sing-a-long. If necessary, refuse to start the car until your child is safely restrained, or pull over to the kerb and adjust the harness each time the child gets out of it. The law requires that you must not travel with your young child unrestrained.

Check that the harness is done up firmly each time you drive. The shoulder straps on a child car seat must be level with, or come from above, your child's shoulders. You will need to move it to a higher level as your child gets taller.

A booster seat is used when a child is too big for the child car seat. A booster seat can be used with a child harness (an H-harness). The harness attaches to the car bolt and the lap belt in the back seat of the car. The booster seat can also be used with an adult lap-sash seat belt, in which case you should use a SafeFit. The SafeFit positions the seat belt correctly on the child's shoulder so that it does not come into contact with the child's neck. When the child is too big for the booster seat, a child harness can be used on its own, or, alternatively, the adult lap-sash seat belt with or without a SafeFit.

Your child is big enough to use an adult seatbelt when the sash part sits flat on the shoulder, and does not touch the child's face or neck.

The following guide will help you decide what type of car restraint you need for your child. Always read the information on the car restraint packaging, including the weight limits.

Child car restraints: types and maximum weights limits (based on the 1995 version of the Australian/New Zealand Standard, AS/NZS 1754: 1995).

Up to 9 kg (and 700 mm long)
Rearward-facing baby restraint
(single-purpose or convertible baby/child restraint)

8 kg   **18 kg**
Forward-facing child car seat
(single-purpose or convertible baby/child restraint)

14 kg   **26 kg**
Booster seat* and a child harness (an H-harness).
Booster seat* and an adult lap-sash seat belt,
with or without a SafeFit.

Up to 32 kg
Child harness (an H-harness) on car seat.
Adult lap-sash seat belt with a SafeFit.

* Used until the child's eye level reaches the top of the booster seat back, or car seat back or headrest.

Safety products

The following safety products and many more are available to buy (including by mail order) from the Safety Centre at the Royal Children's Hospital, Melbourne. For more information and a catalogue, contact the Safety Centre. See **What the Safety Centre can do for you** (p. 146).

Elbow catch: ideal for locking medicines and poisons safely away.

Magnetic lock: a magnetic 'key' is used to open the lock inside a cupboard or drawer.

Safety latch: a plastic latch that must be pressed to open a cupboard or drawer.

Poisons cabinet: metal cabinet (small and large) with a child-resistant elbow catch inside.

Playpen: made of lightweight plastic-coated metal, this can be placed into different shapes or made into a long barrier.

Door or stair barrier: metal barriers or half-doors of varying widths.

Finger-safe guard: clear, thick vinyl that covers door hinges to prevent fingers being jammed in doors.

Curly or coiled cord: keeps a kettle, jug or toaster out of reach of a child.

Stove guard: fits around the top of an upright or benchtop stove to stop children from pulling saucepans down.

Fire blanket or smothering cloth: made from glass fibre, particularly useful for fat and oil fires when water must not be used.

Smoke detector: battery-operated detector, or electric-operated detector with battery back-up are available.

Power-point cover: fits snugly into a power socket.

Heater guard: a range of guards are available for different types of fires and heaters.

Corner cover: made of soft plastic and used on the corners of a table or bench.

Safety checklist

The following list is a general guide only. Leave out those questions that don't apply to you. If you are unsure about any of the safety products, refer to **Safety products** above. If you are unsure about any of the items below (for example, the Australian Standard for nursery furniture), then tick 'Action', as you will need to find out. When you have completed the checklist, summarise what you need to do, and write this in the **Action plan** section at the end of this chapter (p. 19).

In the house

	Yes	No	Action
Emergency numbers by phone	☐	☐	☐
First aid kit available	☐	☐	☐
Completed a child-based first aid resuscitation course	☐	☐	☐
Completed a CPR refresher course in the last year	☐	☐	☐
Chemicals, medicines, cosmetics in locked cupboards	☐	☐	☐
Door of dishwasher kept closed	☐	☐	☐
Smoke detectors installed, and batteries checked	☐	☐	☐
Fire-escape plan practised regularly	☐	☐	☐
Matches and cigarette lighters in locked cupboards	☐	☐	☐
Child-resistant cigarette lighters used	☐	☐	☐
Stove guard fitted	☐	☐	☐
Back burners on the stove used	☐	☐	☐

	Yes	No	Action
Fire blanket or fire extinguisher available	☐	☐	☐
Power-point covers fitted	☐	☐	☐
Safety switches installed	☐	☐	☐
Electrical appliances unplugged after use	☐	☐	☐
Hairdryer and/or electric shaver in locked cupboard	☐	☐	☐
'Low fire danger' children's nightwear chosen	☐	☐	☐
Fireguard or heater guard attached	☐	☐	☐
Curly cord for kettle, jug or toaster	☐	☐	☐
Hot drinks always out of reach of children	☐	☐	☐
Placemats used instead of tablecloth	☐	☐	☐
Temperature control devices or safety taps installed	☐	☐	☐
Household hot water system set to 50–55°C	☐	☐	☐
Door barriers to:			
kitchen	☐	☐	☐
bathroom	☐	☐	☐
laundry	☐	☐	☐
Non-slip surface on bath or non-slip bath mat used	☐	☐	☐
Children in bath always supervised	☐	☐	☐
Nappy bucket off the floor and placed out of reach	☐	☐	☐
Barriers on internal stairs	☐	☐	☐
High chair and change table fitted with body harness	☐	☐	☐
Foods such as hard sweets, carrot, apple, peanuts, popcorn, and food with bones not given to young children	☐	☐	☐
Design of cot meets the Australian Standard	☐	☐	☐
Cot mattress fits snugly	☐	☐	☐
Mobiles, power points, curtain cords kept well away from cot/bed	☐	☐	☐
All blind cords out of reach	☐	☐	☐
Corner covers on sharp edges of furniture	☐	☐	☐
Safety glass or shatter-resistant film on glass	☐	☐	☐
Finger-safe guards on doors	☐	☐	☐
Warning labels on toys checked before buying	☐	☐	☐
Toys in good condition	☐	☐	☐

Outdoors

	Yes	No	Action
Pram or stroller fitted with body harness	☐	☐	☐
Swimming pool surrounded by a fence approved by Standards Australia, with a self-locking, self-latching gate	☐	☐	☐
Wading pool always emptied after use	☐	☐	☐

	Yes	No	Action
Children near water always supervised	☐	☐	☐
A safe fenced area provided for children to play	☐	☐	☐
Fence in good condition	☐	☐	☐
Children encouraged to play in shade, and wear hats and clothing to protect them from the sun	☐	☐	☐
Small amounts of SPF 15+ sunscreen used on hands, feet and face of children	☐	☐	☐
Play equipment in good condition	☐	☐	☐
Soft surface under playground equipment	☐	☐	☐
Children always supervised near dogs	☐	☐	☐
Locked doors on:			
garage	☐	☐	☐
garden shed	☐	☐	☐
Paints and flammable liquids in locked cupboards	☐	☐	☐
Poisonous substances (including pesticides) kept in original containers, and out of reach in locked cupboards	☐	☐	☐
Garden checked for poisonous plants	☐	☐	☐
No tree branches at child's eye level	☐	☐	☐

On the roads

	Yes	No	Action
First aid kit kept in the car	☐	☐	☐
Fire extinguisher kept in the car	☐	☐	☐
Know the correct child restraints approved by Standards Australia to use for your child:			
up to 9 kg	☐	☐	☐
8–18 kg	☐	☐	☐
14–26 kg	☐	☐	☐
up to 32 kg	☐	☐	☐
Child restraints properly fitted	☐	☐	☐
Safety catch on car doors always used	☐	☐	☐
Children always get in and out of the car on the kerbside	☐	☐	☐
Gate to the road kept closed	☐	☐	☐
When near a road, always hold a toddler's hand			
Traffic lights or pedestrian crossing used when available	☐	☐	☐
Understand and know to teach children to 'Stop, Look, Listen, and Think' before and while crossing roads	☐	☐	☐
Children wear a bicycle helmet approved by Standards Australia	☐	☐	☐

Action plan

Photocopy this page, fill it in, and put it on your fridge door as a constant reminder.

What I must do	When	✓
e.g.		
Remove poisons to locked cupboard.	*Immediately*	✓
Find out about Australian Standards on nursery furniture.	*Today*	✓
Buy wood chips for backyard play equipment.	*Saturday*	
Check toys for safety.	*Today*	
Book into a refresher first aid course.	*Phone for information this week*	

Emergencies

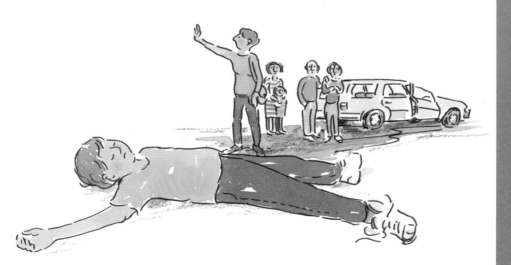

Being prepared for emergencies

'My greatest fear is that I'll forget what to do.'
'What if my mind goes blank, the thought of my child's life
being in my hands scares me.'

Parents and caregivers often express fears about what they would do and how they would react in a life-threatening situation involving a child, particularly their own. The thought of not being able to protect your child from some harm or illness *is* frightening.

In an emergency it is not uncommon to feel a sense of panic, fear, helplessness or confusion. Such feelings are normal responses to an emergency, and felt by even the most experienced first aider and health professional. A little stress can drive a person to act, too much stress can overwhelm you and result in an inability to do anything.

Keeping calm

When you are faced with an emergency, it is important to remain calm and objective. You will need to act quickly but calmly. A child will be fearful and look to you for reassurance; be open and honest, and explain what is happening — the child's imagination may take over, causing further distress.

Emergency phone numbers

The outcome of many emergencies depends upon quick action. Trying to find phone numbers in the white or yellow telephone directories isn't easy when you are in a hurry or feeling anxious. Plan for an emergency, and keep a list of telephone numbers by the phone — on the inside back cover you will find a list of the main emergency numbers you will need to fill in. Copy this page, write in the numbers, and keep it beside the telephone. Write the numbers in your diary too. If you have a touch phone, use the memory dialling facility — of course, in this case you will need to make sure that your toddler doesn't play with the phone.

Let your babysitter know if your child has any illnesses, and what to do in an emergency. Leave your contact number, as well as that of a neighbour.

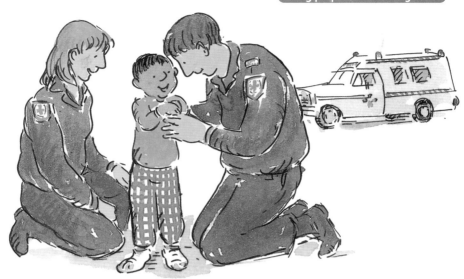

How and when to get medical help

When you no longer feel comfortable dealing with a sick or injured child do not hesitate to call for help. In any emergency always call for an ambulance immediately. Even if you are uncertain about the seriousness of a child's illness or injury, or simply unsure about what to do, call an ambulance. It's better to be over-cautious and allow someone who is trained to deal with emergencies to assess the situation.

A seriously ill or injured child should not be transported to hospital by car. Whenever possible, call an ambulance. Ambulance officers and paramedics can assess, treat and safely transport your child to hospital.

In metropolitan areas and regional centres, simply dial 000, and ask for an ambulance. If you live in the country or an outlying area, the telephone number may be different. Find out the number of your local ambulance service before an emergency occurs, and keep it near your telephone.

When the emergency is over

After an emergency it is sometimes helpful to talk to someone about what has happened. You may feel a sense of relief that the crisis is over, but at the same time you may be upset, unsettled or even overwhelmed. Seek out someone you can talk to. There are professional counsellors who can also help and support you.

First aid courses

Being ready for an emergency helps you to overcome your fears. There are many first aid and resuscitation courses specifically designed for dealing with babies and children. Children are not little adults. It is important that you know the difference in first aid techniques used for children compared to adults.

You may have already completed a course; however, an update is essential at least once a year. Only through practising such skills can you hope to recall them in an emergency. And you will!

Information about first aid courses in your area can be obtained from your local ambulance service or child safety organisation.

First aid kits

It is important to have a first aid kit readily available at home or, when travelling or on holiday, keep one in the car, caravan, boat or in your backpack. You can buy one, or make it yourself. To make a general-purpose first aid kit, you will need to buy the items shown on p. 25 from a chemist's shop or a supermarket, and put them into a large plastic container, fishing-tackle box or poisons cabinet (see **Safety products**, pp. 15–16).

Your first aid kit should contain protective equipment such as rubber gloves and a resuscitation face mask, but never delay first aid and resuscitation if these devices are not available. A resuscitation face mask, such as the Laerdal Pocket Mask, allows you to avoid direct contact with a person's mouth or nose during resuscitation, and reduces the risk of infection. If you are buying a face mask, make sure you have been trained in how to use it, and that it complies with Australian Standard AS4259-1995, 'Ancillary Devices for Expired Air Resuscitation'.

Your first aid kit should contain:

basic first aid notes
pencil and note pad
disposable rubber gloves
resuscitation pocket mask
scissors
safety pins
tweezers (splinter forceps)
individually wrapped sterile adhesive dressings, e.g. Band-Aids
small, medium and large sterile unmedicated wound dressings
sterile non-stick dressing, e.g. Melolin

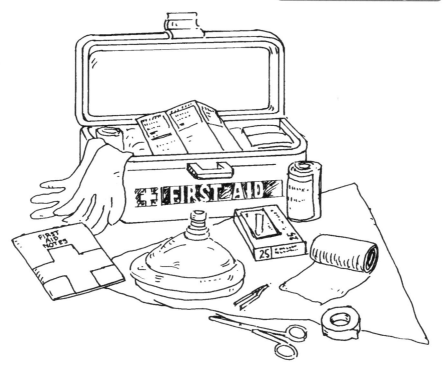

sterile combine dressings
sterile cotton gauze swabs (7.5 cm x 7.5 cm)
adhesive tape (2.5 cm)
triangular bandages
stretch bandages (5 cm, 7.5 cm, 10 cm)
sterile eye pads
antiseptic solution, e.g. Betadine
sterile normal saline solution, e.g. Eyestream
anti-irritant solution for bites and stings, e.g. Stingose
individual plastic bags
disposable aluminium foil banket (available from outdoor and camping
    shops)

If the items for your first aid kit are not available, make use of other
common household materials mentioned throughout the book.

Life-threatening emergencies

The ABC of caring for a child until an ambulance arrives

In a life-threatening emergency your quick and clear thinking is essential. The more you are prepared for an emergency, the easier it will be to remember what to do. Enrol in a child-based resuscitation class, keep the **resuscitation chart** (front flap) handy, and reread this chapter regularly.

All life-threatening emergencies should be treated in the same way. You need to follow certain steps, which are easy to remember if you say to yourself 'A B C':

> **A** is for **AIRWAY**
> **B** is for **BREATHING**
> **C** is for **CIRCULATION.**

The **Life-threatening emergencies chart** (front flap) summarises the main steps to follow. These steps are explained in more detail below.

Some of the techniques differ depending upon the age of the child — a baby (under 1 year), a small child (approximately 1–8 years) or a large child (approximately over 8 years). Where necessary, these differences will be pointed out, otherwise any reference in this chapter made to 'child' will include a child of any age, including a baby.

Make the area safe

1. *If you can, remove or move away from any hazards that may put you or the child at further risk; for example, from electricity or traffic.*

2. *Call for an ambulance. If necessary, ask someone to get help from the police, fire brigade, state emergency service or other rescue service, or to redirect traffic.*

3. *If necessary, gently move the child to a safer area.*

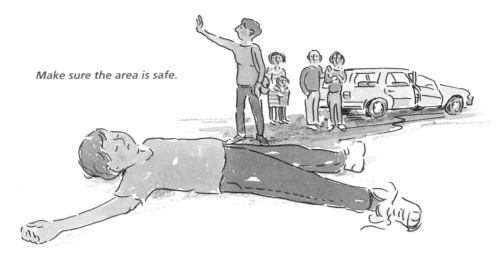

Make sure the area is safe.

Check if the child is conscious or unconscious

1 *Shake the child firmly by the shoulders, and shout loudly into the ear.*

2 *Ask the child to squeeze your hand.*

3 *If there is no response, the child is unconscious.*

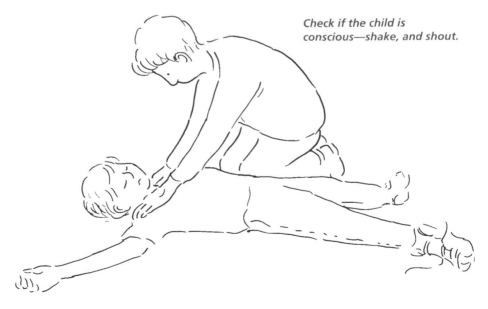

Check if the child is conscious—shake, and shout.

Place child on one side.

An unconscious child MUST ALWAYS be placed on one side with the head turned slightly downwards. This protects the airway from becoming blocked by the tongue, blood or vomit. If an unconscious child has other injuries such as fractures, the child must still be placed on one side. Try to move the child as gently as possible, supporting any injured limbs, and ask other people to help.

Airway

1 *With the child lying on one side, gently scoop away any material from the entrance of the mouth with your fingers. Clear a baby's nose by gently squeezing it.*

Baby: slightly lift jaw — no head tilt.

2 *Open the child's airway by tilting back the head and lifting the chin. The amount of head tilt depends on the size and age of the child.*

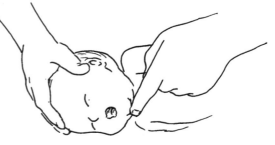

28

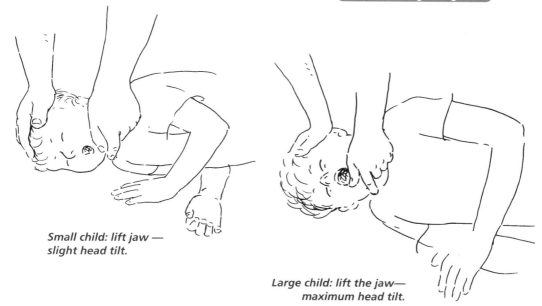

*Small child: lift jaw —
slight head tilt.*

*Large child: lift the jaw—
maximum head tilt.*

Breathing

1 **Check if the child is breathing by:**
• looking for the rise and fall of the chest and stomach
• listening and feeling for air from the mouth and nose.

2 **If the child is breathing, leave the child lying on one side.
Recheck the breathing every minute, and stay with the child
until the ambulance arrives.**
**If the child is not breathing, you will need to breathe for the
child. This is known as *mouth-to-mouth resuscitation.***

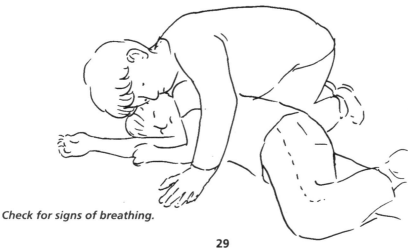

Check for signs of breathing.

29

Mouth-to-mouth resuscitation

Baby

1 *Carefully roll the baby onto its back.*

2 *Open the airway (see AIRWAY above).*

3 *Open the baby's mouth slightly, and cover the mouth and nose with your mouth. Alternatively, cover the nose only, in which case the baby's mouth should be closed.*

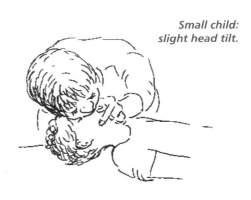

Baby: no head tilt.

4 *Give 5 gentle puffs from your cheeks in 10 seconds. Only blow until the chest starts to rise. If the chest does not rise, recheck the head tilt and jaw lift, and try again.*
    Then proceed with steps 6–9 on p. 31.

Small or large child

1 *Carefully roll the child onto its back.*

2 *Open the airway (see AIRWAY above).*

3 *Block the nose with your cheek, or pinch it closed.*

4 *Open the child's mouth slightly, and cover it with your mouth.*

Small child: slight head tilt.

5 *Give 5 gentle breaths in 10 seconds. Only blow until the chest starts to rise. If the chest does not rise, recheck the head tilt and jaw lift, and try again.*

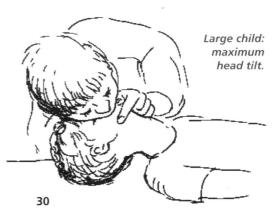

Large child: maximum head tilt.

6 **After the first 5 breaths feel for the pulse in the child's neck over 5 seconds.**

7 **If the child has a pulse but is not breathing,** *continue mouth-to-mouth resuscitation, as below.* **If you cannot feel a pulse,** *go to* CIRCULATION.

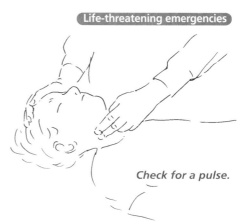

Check for a pulse.

Mouth-to-mouth resuscitation breathing rates

Baby :   1 gentle puff every 3 seconds.
Small child: 1 gentle breath every 3 seconds.
Large child: 1 full breath every 4 seconds.

8 **Recheck the pulse and breathing after 1 minute, and then every 2 minutes.**

9 **Continue breathing for the child until the child starts to breathe, or until an ambulance arrives. If the child starts to breathe, place the child on one side, and continue to regularly check the breathing and pulse.**

Circulation

If the child **is unconscious, not breathing and has no pulse, then start cardiopulmonary resuscitation (CPR).** CPR combines mouth-to-mouth resuscitation with chest compressions. It can be done by one person alone or by two people working together. When on your own, you will need to breathe for the child and compress (push down on) the chest. When there are two people, take turns: one breathes for the child, then rests while the other compresses the chest.

CPR can keep the blood and oxygen circulating until an ambulance arrives, and sometimes restarts the child's heart.

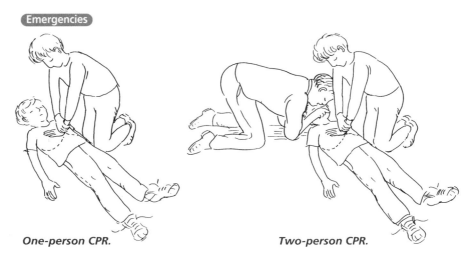

One-person CPR.   Two-person CPR.

Cardiopulmonary resuscitation (CPR)

Don't be frightened to try. You have nothing to lose, and you are giving the child a chance of survival. Remind yourself that you have the ability, knowledge and skills to help the child.

Locate the lower half of the breastbone of the child, as shown. Make sure you don't press below the bottom of the breastbone.

Baby

1 *Place two fingers on the lower half of the breastbone. Gently press down about 2 cm only.*
Then proceed with steps 2–5 on p. 34.

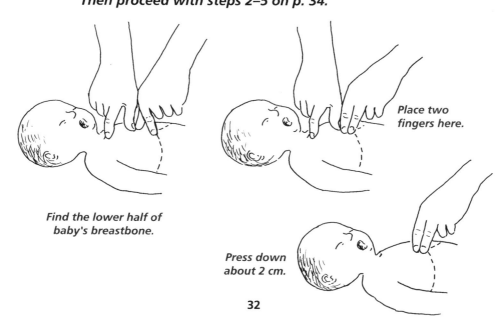

Find the lower half of baby's breastbone.

Place two fingers here.

Press down about 2 cm.

One person	Two people
Give 15 compressions, then 2 gentle puffs, every 10 seconds.	One to give 5 compressions, the other to give 1 gentle puff, every 3 seconds.

Small child

1 *Place heel of one hand on lower half of breastbone. Press down about 3 cm.*
Then proceed with steps 2–5 on p. 34.

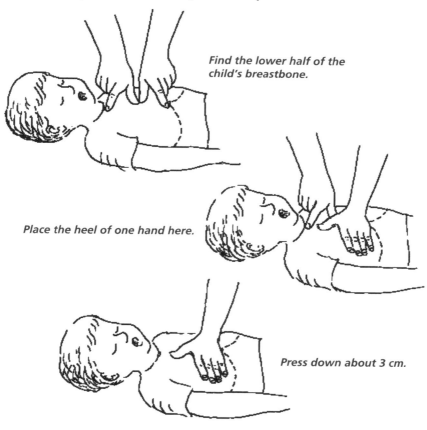

Find the lower half of the child's breastbone.

Place the heel of one hand here.

Press down about 3 cm.

One person	Two people
Give 15 compressions, then 2 breaths, every 10 seconds.	One to give 5 compressions, the other to give 1 gentle breath every 3 seconds.

33

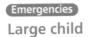

Large child

1 *Place the heel of one hand on the lower half of the breastbone, and grip your wrist with the other hand. Press down about 4-5 cm.*

Find the lower half of the child's breastbone.

Place the heel of one hand here.

Grip with the other hand, and press down about 4–5 cm.

One person	Two people
Give 15 compressions, then 2 breaths, every 15 seconds.	One to give 5 compressions, the other to give 1 breath, every 5 seconds.

2 *Check the child's pulse and breathing after 1 minute of CPR, and then every 2 minutes.*

3 *If the child vomits, place the child on one side. Clear the airway, and continue resuscitation.*

4 *If the child's pulse returns but the child is not breathing, continue mouth-to-mouth resuscitation.*

5 *If the pulse and breathing return, place the child on one side and open the airway. Keep checking the pulse and breathing every 2 minutes until the ambulance arrives.*

34

Injuries

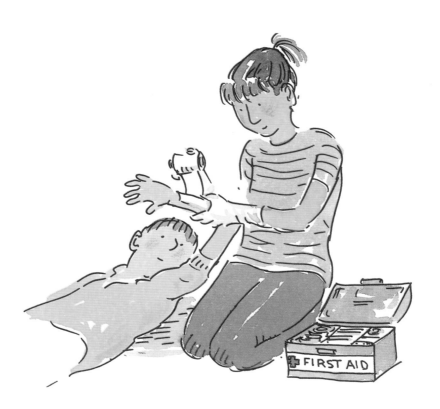

Bites and stings

Facts

Venomous creatures

Australia has many venomous or poisonous creatures. These include bees, wasps, spiders, snakes, ants, bush ticks, and marine or sea animals. It is reassuring to know that there are excellent Australian anti-venoms available for bites from many of these venomous animals.

A bee will sting only once. European wasps are more aggressive than native wasps, and can sting repeatedly — as can ants — and they have been spreading slowly throughout south-eastern Australia. Bee, wasp and ant stings can be painful, but they aren't usually serious unless the child has an allergic reaction or is stung in or around the mouth. See **First aid: Allergic reaction** (p. 40).

There are over 100 species of snakes in Australia, a quarter of which are deadly. Some of the dangerous ones include the taipan, the death adder, and tiger, black, brown and copperhead snakes. Most bites are to the leg or arm.

Of all the spiders, only the funnel-web and the red-back are dangerous to humans. A bite from a white-tailed spider can occasionally cause the skin to blister and ulcerate, but isn't life-threatening.

Marine animal bites and stings are less common, particularly jellyfish stings, but usually are not serious. Some, however, can rapidly become life-threatening. See **Life-threatening emergencies** (pp. 26–34). Australia has some of the most venomous sea creatures in the world, including the box jellyfish, the blue-ringed octopus, the stonefish and the cone shell.

Dogs

Children most at risk of dog bites are under 5 years of age. They are more likely to be bitten by a familiar dog in their own or a friend's home than by an unleashed dog on the street.

The breeds involved in most attacks are bull-terrier, Rottweiler, Dobermann, German shepherd, blue heeler, and border collie. However, potentially all dogs, regardless of breed, can bite. This includes the trusty and faithful old Labrador, especially if a child stands on its tail and gives it a fright.

Because of height, a child is often bitten on the head, face or neck. There is

the possibility of infection, long-term scarring, disfigurement, and in more
serious and savage attacks even death.

Prevention

Venomous creatures

During summer and spring, and in the case of European wasps during spring
to autumn, the risk of children being stung or bitten increases as creatures
become active and children play outside more.

- Children need to develop a healthy
  respect for venomous creatures. Teach
  them not to disturb or provoke these
  creatures, as they are likely to attack.
- Cut the grass regularly, and remove
  rubbish from the front and back yards.

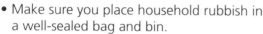

- Make sure you place household rubbish in
  a well-sealed bag and bin.
- Soft drinks from a can or bottle should be
  drunk through a straw, as wasps and bees
  attracted to sweetness hide in the can or
  bottle and can sting the child's mouth and
  throat.
- Keep children well away from a wasp nest.
  Contact your local council, pest control
  company or your state Department of
  Agriculture for help in removing the nest.
- If your child is known to be allergic to bees,
  wasps or ants, make sure the child wears a
  medical-alert bracelet. Children are
  sometimes prescribed medication to
  treat a severe allergic reaction, so
  make sure you or any other carer,
  or an older child, carry the
  medication and know how to
  use it in an emergency.

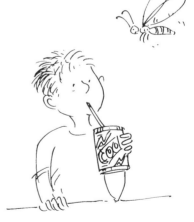

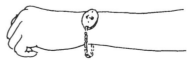

Medical-alert bracelet.

- Use insect repellents on children over 12 months.
- Leave snakes alone! Many children and adults are bitten while trying to kill snakes.
- Children should wear closed-in footwear and long trousers if walking along tracks or in bushland.
- Discourage children from putting their hands into hollow logs or under wood piles.

Children love to play in rock pools at the beach.

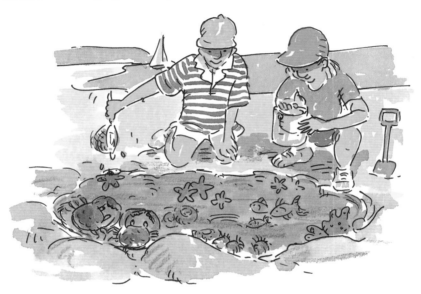

- Warn them of the dangers of picking up empty bottles and cans, lifting rocks or putting shells into their pockets, as some marine animals make them their home. Children need to wear closed-in shoes, such as runners or sandshoes, when exploring.
- The blue-ringed octopus is a tiny creature, normally yellow-brown in colour with dark-blue rings. If the octopus is teased or provoked, the rings turn bright blue, and the octopus will bite. Children can be attracted to its bright colour, and they should be taught never to touch the creature.
- Stay out of tropical waters during October to May when box jellyfish can be active. Remember that there is still a risk at other times of the year. Look for warning signs, and allow children to swim only in patrolled water protected by stinger nets. Specially designed 'stinger' lycra suits, diving wetsuits, or even at a pinch pantyhose, provide some protection. Carry vinegar as part of your first aid kit when you're going to a tropical beach. See **First aid: Box jellyfish** (p. 47).

Dogs

Owning and caring for a family pet can be a wonderful experience for a child.

Some people choose to delay buying a dog until children are older and able to appreciate it more fully. Remember, many a deceptively small and cuddly puppy has grown into a *big*, furry friend!

When buying a dog, consider the breed, temperament and adult size of the dog and, most importantly, the ages and maturity of the children. Wait until the children are at least 4 or 5 years old before buying a dog, as this reduces the chances of head and facial injuries should a dog bite, as the children are taller.

A well-trained, obedient dog that is respectful of its owners is also less likely to be badly behaved or hard to control around children. Consider your ability to train a dog before buying one. Take the dog to obedience classes.

Teach children to pat the back or side of a dog's body, not the head as it may feel threatened. Children must understand that not all dogs are friendly. They should be taught to ask the owner before patting a dog.

When there is already a dog in the household:

- Be aware that the dog may become jealous of a newborn child; keep them separated, and give the dog plenty of attention and affection.
- Teach children to respect and play safely with their dog. If any dog is tormented, it will become defensive. Children must be taught that hitting and teasing are unacceptable. Rough, active play can also over-excite a dog, and it may bite.
- Children should be taught not to disturb a dog while it is eating or sleeping.

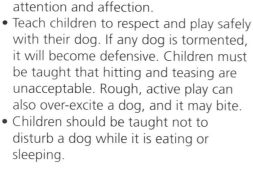
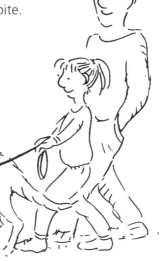

First aid

Allergic reaction

This may occur within seconds or minutes following a bite or sting usually from bees, wasps or some ants. It can be life-threatening.

What to look for

➤ blotchy and itchy rash
➤ face and neck starts to swell
➤ tightness in the chest
➤ wheezing and difficulty in breathing
➤ nausea and vomiting
➤ collapse.

What to do

1   *Calm the child, and keep the child still.*

2   *Put a pressure bandage and splint over the bite area, and call an ambulance.*
   • *Put pressure over the bite using your hands.*
   • *If the child is bitten on a limb, wrap a crepe bandage over the area. If you don't have one, tear some cloth into strips 10–15 cm wide. Bandage upwards from the fingers or toes to cover as much of the arm or leg as possible. It should be firm but not too tight, and can be wrapped over clothing.*
   • *Keep the limb still by using a splint (a piece of wood, umbrella or rolled-up newspaper), if available. Place the child's arm in a sling, or tie the child's legs together.*
   • *Keep the child still. Leave the bandage and splint on until the child reaches hospital.*
   *See **Pressure bandage and splint** (p. 41).*

3   *If the child has prescribed medication for an allergic reaction, help the child to use it immediately.*

4   *If the child becomes unconscious while you are waiting for the ambulance, follow the **Life-threatening emergencies chart** (front flap) until the ambulance arrives.*

Pressure bandage and splint

This stops venom or poison reaching the bloodstream. It is used for many types of bites, and also allergic reactions to a bite or sting.

What to do

1   *Put pressure over the bite, using your hands. Do not wash the area if the child is bitten by a snake.*

2   *If the child is bitten on a limb, wrap a crepe bandage over the bitten area. If you don't have one, tear some cloth into strips 10–15 cm wide. Bandage upwards from the fingers or toes to cover as much of the arm or leg as possible. It should be firm but not too tight, and can be wrapped over clothing.*

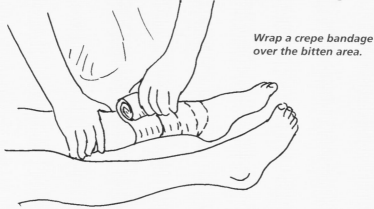

Wrap a crepe bandage over the bitten area.

3   *Keep the limb still by using a splint (a piece of wood, umbrella or rolled-up newspaper), if available. Place the child's arm in a sling, or tie the child's legs together.*

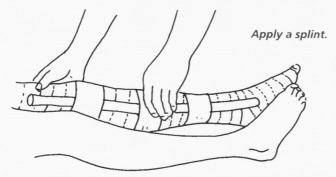

Apply a splint.

4   *Keep the child still. Leave the bandage and splint on until the child reaches hospital.*

Bee, wasp and ant stings

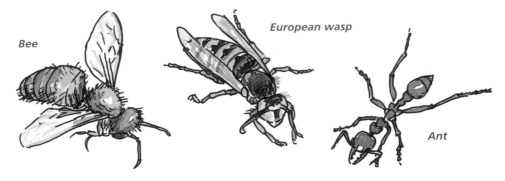

Bee

European wasp

Ant

What to look for
➤ severe pain around sting
➤ redness and swelling.

What to do

1 *Calm the child, and keep the child still.*

2 *If the child is stung by a bee, remove the sting by flicking it off with a fingernail or the edge of a knife. Do not squeeze the area. Unlike bees, wasps don't leave stings.*

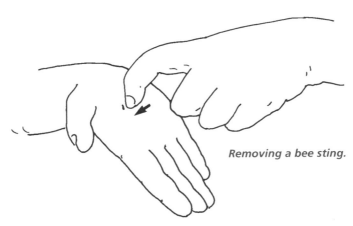

Removing a bee sting.

3 *Wrap some ice in a wet cloth, and put it on the stung area.*

4 *If pain and swelling persist, take the child to a doctor.*

5 If the child is stung in or around the mouth, give the child an ice cube or icypole to suck, and immediately call an ambulance.

6 Watch closely for an allergic reaction. See **Allergic reaction (p. 40)**. If the child has an allergic reaction and the bite is on the arm or leg, use a **pressure bandage and splint** (see p. 41), and call an ambulance.
- Put pressure over the bite using your hands.
- If the child is bitten on a limb, wrap a crepe bandage over the area. If you don't have one, tear some cloth into strips 10–15 cm wide. Bandage upwards from the fingers or toes to cover as much of the arm or leg as possible. It should be firm but not too tight, and can be wrapped over clothing.
- Keep the limb still by using a splint (a piece of wood, umbrella or rolled-up newspaper), if available. Place the child's arm in a sling, or tie the child's legs together.
- Keep the child still. Leave the bandage and splint on until the child reaches hospital.

Funnel-web spider bite

Funnel-web spiders are found mainly in Sydney, coastal NSW and south-east Queensland. Within 10 minutes of a bite a child can be dangerously ill. Any bite from a large black or reddish-brown hairy spider, particularly in the Sydney area, is best treated as if it were from a funnel-web spider.

What to look for

➤ severe pain around the bite
➤ tingling around the mouth
➤ saliva from the mouth
➤ twitching of muscles
➤ difficulty in breathing
➤ stomach pain
➤ sweating
➤ confusion.

Funnel-web spider

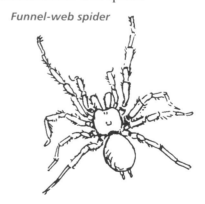

What to do

1 Calm the child, and keep the child still.

2 Put a **pressure bandage and splint** (see p. 41) over the bite area, and call an ambulance.

- *Put pressure over the bite using your hands.*
- *If the child is bitten on a limb, wrap a crepe bandage over the area. If you don't have one, tear some cloth into strips 10–15 cm wide. Bandage upwards from the fingers or toes to cover as much of the arm or leg as possible. It should be firm but not too tight, and can be wrapped over clothing.*
- *Keep the limb still by using a splint (a piece of wood, umbrella or rolled-up newspaper), if available. Place the child's arm in a sling, or tie the child's legs together.*
- *Keep the child still. Leave the bandage and splint on until the child reaches hospital.*

3 *If the child becomes unconscious while you are waiting for the ambulance, follow the **Life-threatening emergencies chart** (front flap) until the ambulance arrives.*

Red-back spider bite

Red-back spiders are found throughout Australia, and a bite from one can be life-threatening. The poison is slow to act, and serious illness rarely happens in under 3 hours.

What to look for
➤ pain around the bite that increases and spreads
➤ redness and swelling around the bite
➤ nausea and vomiting
➤ stomach pain
➤ sweating, particularly around the bite
➤ swollen and sore glands in the armpits or groin
➤ shivering and shaking.

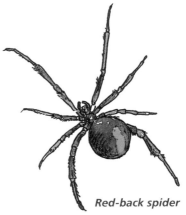
Red-back spider

What to do

1 *Calm the child, and keep the child still.*

2 *Wrap some ice in a wet cloth, and put it on the bite. As red-back spider venom is slow moving, a pressure bandage and splint are not necessary, and will only make the pain worse.*

3 *Call an ambulance.*

44

4 *If the child becomes unconscious while you are waiting, follow the **Life-threatening emergencies chart** (front flap) until the ambulance arrives.*

Snake bite

Life-threatening effects from a snake bite usually aren't seen for a few hours, but can sometimes appear in minutes.

What to look for
➤ fang marks
➤ headache and blurred vision
➤ difficulty in speaking, swallowing or breathing
➤ nausea and vomiting
➤ stomach pain
➤ swollen glands in the armpits or groin
➤ weakness
➤ collapse.

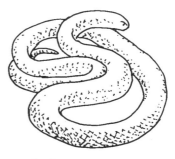

Snake

What to do

1 *Calm the child, and keep the child still.*

2 *Don't cut, wash or suck the bite, or use a tourniquet.*

3 *Put a **pressure bandage and splint** (see p. 41) over the bite area, and call an ambulance.*
• *Put pressure over the bite using your hands.*
• *If the child is bitten on a limb, wrap a crepe bandage over the area. If you don't have one, tear some cloth into strips 10–15 cm wide. Bandage upwards from the fingers or toes to cover as much of the arm or leg as possible. It should be firm but not too tight, and can be wrapped over clothing.*
• *Keep the limb still by using a splint (a piece of wood, umbrella or rolled-up newspaper), if available. Place the child's arm in a sling, or tie the child's legs together.*
• *Keep the child still. Leave the bandage and splint on until the child reaches hospital.*

4 *If the child becomes unconscious while you are waiting for the ambulance, follow the **Life-threatening emergencies chart** (front flap) until the ambulance arrives.*

Bush tick bite

The bush tick is a small insect found mainly along the eastern coast of Australia, from Queensland to northern Tasmania. A bite can cause paralysis. Symptoms usually show up over a few days, but allergic reactions can happen in a few hours.

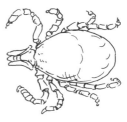

Bush tick

What to look for
➤ itching, redness, swelling or pain around the bite
➤ the child is unsteady on feet
➤ tiredness and muscle weakness
➤ double vision
➤ difficulty breathing or swallowing.

What to do

1 *Find the tick. A tick can be anywhere on the body, but it prefers hairy areas, skin creases and ears.*

2 *Gently lever or slowly pull the tick out, using sharp-pointed tweezers placed as close as possible to the mouth-parts of the tick. Don't squeeze the area, as more venom may be injected, or part of the tick may be left under the skin.*

3 *Take the child to a doctor as soon as possible.*

4 *Sometimes a tick bite may cause an allergic reaction (see **Allergic reaction**, p. 40). If this occurs, and the bite is on the arm or leg, use **a pressure bandage and splint** (see p. 41), and call an ambulance.*
   * *Put pressure over the bite using your hands.*
   * *If the child is bitten on a limb, wrap a crepe bandage over the area. If you don't have one, tear some cloth into strips 10–15 cm wide. Bandage upwards from the fingers or toes to cover as much of the arm or leg as possible. It should be firm but not too tight, and can be wrapped over clothing.*
   * *Keep the limb still by using a splint (a piece of wood, umbrella or rolled-up newspaper), if available. Place the child's arm in a sling, or tie the child's legs together.*
   * *Keep the child still. Leave the bandage and splint on until the child reaches hospital.*

5 *If the child becomes unconscious while you are waiting for the ambulance, follow the **Life-threatening emergencies chart** (front flap) until the ambulance arrives.*

Box jellyfish sting

All jellyfish have tentacles that cause pain upon skin contact. Only those jellyfish in tropical northern Australia, such as the box jellyfish, are deadly. If stung, a child can die in minutes.

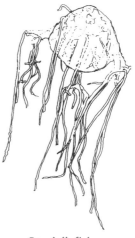

Box jellyfish

What to look for
➤ immediate, severe burning pain
➤ swollen and purplish red lines (like whip marks) around the bitten area
➤ tentacles sticking to the skin
➤ the child becomes irrational
➤ unconsciousness
➤ the child stops breathing, and has no pulse.

What to do

1 *Remove the child from the water. Calm the child, and keep the child still. Stop the child from rubbing the sting.*

2 *If the child becomes unconscious, follow the **Life-threatening emergencies chart** (front flap) while treating the sting.*

3 *Call an ambulance.*

4 *If it is available, pour plenty of vinegar over the sting to stop the tentacles from releasing further venom into the skin. If vinegar isn't available, pinch off any tentacles with your fingers.*

5 *If it is a minor sting, wrap some ice in a wet cloth and put it on the sting to help ease any pain.*

6 *If the sting covers a large area (half or more of a limb), put a pressure bandage and splint over the treated area, as follows.*
 • *Do not bandage any area that has not been treated with vinegar or had the tentacles removed, as more venom may be released into the skin.*

47

• *Using a crepe bandage, or some cloth torn into strips 10–15 cm wide, bandage upwards from the fingers or toes to cover as much of the arm or leg as possible. The bandage should be firm, but not too tight. Pour more vinegar over the bandage.*

7 *Keep the limb still by using a splint (a piece of wood, umbrella or rolled-up newspaper), if available. Place the child's arm in a sling, or tie the child's legs together. Leave the bandage and splint on until the child reaches hospital. Note: Vinegar should be used only for box jellyfish stings.*

Bluebottle jellyfish sting

The bluebottle jellyfish is found around the whole coastline of Australia. It can cause a painful sting; however, this is rarely life-threatening.

What to look for
➤ skin pain
➤ skin welts (often white with red edges)
➤ pain in the armpits or groin
➤ nausea or vomiting
➤ headache
➤ the child may be drowsy if it is a major sting.

Bluebottle jellyfish

What to do

1 *Remove the child from the water. Calm the child, and keep the child still. Stop the child from rubbing the sting.*

2 *Wash off any fresh tentacles with seawater. If it is a minor sting, wrap some ice in a dry cloth, and put it on the sting for at least 10–15 minutes to reduce the pain. If the pain continues, keep applying ice, wrapped in a dry cloth.*

3 *If the child's condition doesn't improve, call an ambulance.*

4 *If the child becomes unconscious while you are waiting for the ambulance, follow the **Life-threatening emergencies chart** (front flap) until the ambulance arrives.*

Blue-ringed octopus and cone shell stings

The blue-ringed octopus is found in all Australian coastal waters and beaches, the cone shell has a snail-like creature inside that can sting; it is found in tropical waters. Both the blue-ringed octopus and the cone shell are highly venomous. Their bite or sting is almost painless, and it may not be obvious that a child has been bitten until becoming ill. A serious bite or sting can result in death within 30 minutes if not treated.

What to look for
➤ a spot of blood around the bite
➤ lips and tongue become numb
➤ difficulty in swallowing
➤ breathing difficulties
➤ the child may stop breathing.

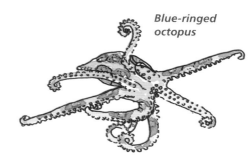

Blue-ringed octopus

What to do

1   **Calm the child, and keep the child still.**

2   **Put a pressure bandage and splint (see p. 41) over the sting, and call an ambulance.**

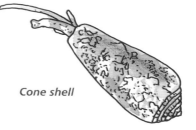

Cone shell

   • **Put pressure over the bite using your hands.**
   • **If the child is bitten on a limb, wrap a crepe bandage over the area. If you don't have one, tear some cloth into strips 10–15 cm wide. Bandage upwards from the fingers or toes to cover as much of the arm or leg as possible. It should be firm but not too tight, and can be wrapped over clothing.**
   • **Keep the limb still by using a splint (a piece of wood, umbrella or rolled-up newspaper), if available. Place the child's arm in a sling, or tie the child's legs together.**
   • **Keep the child still. Leave the bandage and splint on until the child reaches hospital.**

3   **If the child becomes unconscious while you are waiting for the ambulance, follow the Life-threatening emergencies chart (front flap) until the ambulance arrives.**

Stonefish, bullrout and stingray stings

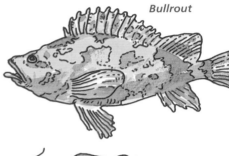

Stonefish

Stonefish (in seawater) and bullrouts (in fresh water) are found in tropical waters, coral reefs and beaches. They can be mistaken for rocks, and a child can be stung when picking them up or standing on them. Their sting can cause severe pain but is rarely life-threatening.

Stingrays are found around the whole coast of Australia, and have a whip-like tail that can cause a painful and deep wound.

Bullrout

What to look for
➤ an open wound and bleeding
➤ severe spreading pain
➤ stung area swells, and may change to a greyish-blue colour
➤ irrational behaviour.

What to do

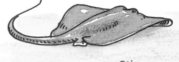

Stingray

1 **Calm the child, and keep the child still.**

2 **If possible, place the stung arm or leg in warm to hot water to inactivate the venom. Check the temperature first to make sure it isn't too hot, as it may burn the child.**

3 **Do not bandage the wound.**

4 **Call an ambulance.**

5 **If the child becomes unconscious while you are waiting for the ambulance, follow the Life-threatening emergencies chart (front flap) until the ambulance arrives.**

Dog bites

What to do

1 **Calm and reassure the child.**

2 Dog bites can cause infection. If the skin has been broken, wash the area under cold running water.

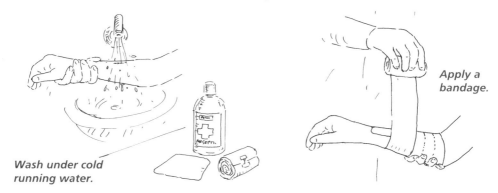

Wash under cold running water.

Apply a bandage.

3 Apply antiseptic, and cover the bite with a clean dressing or cloth. Take the child to a doctor for a tetanus booster and antibiotics, if necessary.

4 If a piece of flesh or body part has been bitten off:
- Try not to panic. Calm and reassure the child. Most amputated parts can be reattached successfully with surgery.
- Call an ambulance.
- Control any bleeding by applying firm pressure to the wound using a sterile dressing, clean cloth, towel or other bulky material. If possible, hold the injured part up high, preferably above the child's chest height.
- Keep the dressing in place by wrapping a bandage firmly around it. Make sure it is not too tight—there should be no tingling or throbbing. If necessary, loosen the bandage but do not remove the dressing.
- If the bleeding continues, put another dressing on top and wrap another firm bandage around it. Keep applying pressure with your hands around the wound.
- If the child is pale or drowsy, the child may be in shock. Lie the child down, and raise the legs on a folded blanket or pillow. Keep the child warm with a blanket or coat, being careful not to overheat. If the child is thirsty, wet the lips with a wet facewasher or cloth. Do not give any food or water. For more information see **Shock** (p. 55).
- Gently place the amputated part in a clean plastic bag, and seal the bag.
- Place the sealed bag in a container filled with water and a few ice cubes. Do not let the body part come in direct contact with the ice, as it can cause damage.
- Keep reassuring the child until the ambulance arrives.

Bleeding

Facts

Cuts, 'skinned' knees and scrapes often result from falls at home. Children are sometimes injured when playing too close to low windows and glass doors, from falling from play equipment, or simply running and falling in the backyard. An increasing number of children have suffered severe finger injuries as a result of fingers being jammed in door hinges, or caught in the chains and wheels of exercise bikes.

It is important to control all bleeding as quickly as possible, especially in children. The amount of blood in a person's body depends on their weight and size: an average adult has about 6 litres, a 2-year-old child has about 1 litre.

Whereas an adult can give 500 ml of blood as a donation, a child losing this amount of blood will become seriously ill. Because of smaller body size, a child may go into shock if too much blood is lost. See **Shock** (p. 55).

The body has its own way of stopping bleeding. Blood vessels constrict around the cut or wound; this slows down the flow of blood to the area, and allows a clot to form. First aid treatment will assist the body in this process.

Prevention

In their attempts to stand, babies will grab on to furniture for support. They will be unsteady, and will fall suddenly and often.

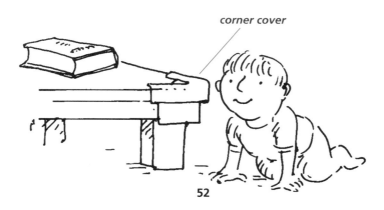

corner cover

- Remove any glass-topped table, and store it until your child is older.
- Protect table corners with plastic corner covers. See **Safety products** (pp. 15–16).

Active and curious toddlers will run and jump about with increasing speed and risk.

- Place sharp knives, glass jars, bottles and drinking glasses in cupboards with child-resistant locks. See **Safety products**.
- A child should sit down while eating, and should use plastic eating utensils.
- Discourage children from walking or running around with glass or sharp objects.
- Apply shatter-resistant film (a special type of clear plastic film) to low-lying unprotected glass (glass that is not laminated or toughened); for example, on windows, doors and glass-topped tables.
- Put brightly coloured stickers or transfers on these glass surfaces to remind children of their presence.
- Place furniture in front of glass doors and floor-length windows to create a barrier.
- Install a door closure to slow down the speed of a closing door.
- Place finger guards on the hinge side of doors. See **Safety products**.
- Install a door stopper (a rubber device that hooks over the top of the door) to stop the door from closing completely.
- If you are buying an exercise bike, make sure it has a solid wheel and a safety cover over the chain and wheels. If you have a bike without these, put a lock on the wheels and pedals to stop them from moving. Keep young children away from the bike at all times.
- Lock away tools and machinery. Never allow a child to ride on a tractor or ride-on mower.
- Avoid buying toys made from brittle plastic or with sharp edges. Check older toys for signs of damage, such as broken plastic or splintered wood.

First aid

WARNING

Always treat blood as possibly infectious. Wherever possible, wear tight, disposable rubber gloves. If these are not available, use a plastic bag over your hand, or other similar material. If you come into contact with blood, wash it off immediately with soap and water.

Many children are frightened by the sight of blood, and need to be reassured. Aim to cover the wound as quickly as possible. If you have one available, use a red or dark-coloured facewasher or hand towel.

Minor wound

What to do

1 *Clean any minor wound with soap and water.*

2 *Apply an antiseptic solution, and a clean dressing.*

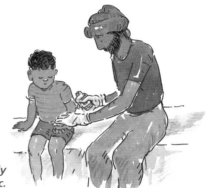

After cleaning the wound, apply an antiseptic.

Major wound

What to do

1 *Lie the child down. Calm the child, and keep the child still.*

2 *If an arm or leg has been injured and is bleeding, hold it up as high as possible, preferably above the child's chest height. This slows down the blood supply to the wound.*

Hold the bleeding limb up high.

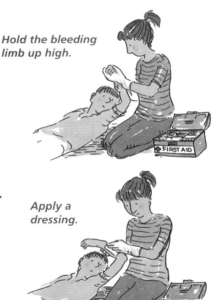

3 *If nothing is stuck in the wound, apply firm pressure, using a sterile dressing, clean cloth, towel or other bulky material. If there is something stuck in the wound, see **Foreign body** (p. 56).*

Apply a dressing.

4 *Keep the dressing in place by wrapping a bandage firmly around it. Make sure it is not too tight; there should be no tingling or throbbing. If it is too tight, loosen the bandage but don't remove the dressing.*

Apply a bandage.

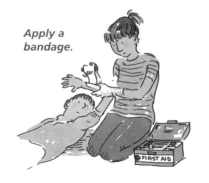

5   *If the bleeding continues, put another dressing on top and wrap another firm bandage around it. Apply pressure with your hands around the wound. Keep doing this until the bleeding stops.*

6   *If the cut is serious, take the child to a doctor.*

7   *If the bleeding can't be stopped or the child has lost a lot of blood, is drowsy or pale, call an ambulance. See **Shock** below.*

Shock

A child who has lost a large amount of blood may go into shock. Shock may also be caused by burns, prolonged vomiting and diarrhoea, severe fractures or amputation. Shock can be life-threatening, and must be recognised and treated urgently.

What to look for
➤ pale, cool skin (older children may sweat)
➤ fast pulse
➤ fast, shallow breathing
➤ dizziness
➤ drowsiness and weakness
➤ vomiting.

What to do

1   *Calm and reassure the child, and lie the child down.*

2   *Raise the legs, using a pillow, a rolled-up blanket, towels or other bulky materials.*

3   *Keep treating the injury or illness that is the cause of shock, and call an ambulance.*

4   *Keep the child warm with a blanket or coat. Be careful not to overheat the child, as this may make the shock worse.*

5   *If the child is thirsty, wet the lips with a wet facewasher or cloth. Do not give any food or water in case the child becomes unconscious or requires an anaesthetic.*

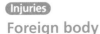
Foreign body

Minor wound
What to do

1 **Remove any gravel and dirt with a wet cloth or hold the wound under running water, if possible, until clean.**

Object stuck in the wound
What to do

If something larger is deeply stuck in the wound, do not attempt to remove it.

1 **Calm the child, and lie the child down.**

2 **Control the bleeding around the object by gently pressing the edges of the wound together.**

3 **Build up dressings around the object, and keep them in place with a bandage wrapped diagonally.**

4 **Take the child immediately to a doctor or a hospital emergency department. If the foreign body is large, or the child is pale or drowsy, call an ambulance.**

5 **If the child is pale or drowsy, raise the legs with a pillow or folded blanket. See Shock (p. 55) for further information.**

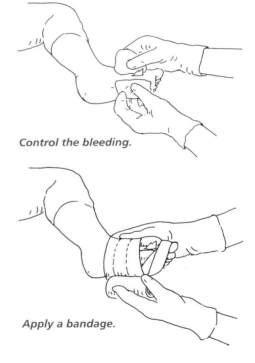

Control the bleeding.

Apply a bandage.

Amputation

What to do

Treat as for a major wound. See pp. 54–5.

1 **Try not to panic. Calm and reassure the child. Most amputated parts can be successfully reattached with surgery.**

2 Control any bleeding by applying firm pressure to the wound using a sterile dressing, clean cloth, towel or other bulky material. If possible, hold the injured part up high, preferably above the child's chest height.

3 Call an ambulance.

4 Keep the dressing in place by wrapping a bandage firmly around it. Make sure it is not too tight — there should be no tingling or throbbing. If necessary, loosen the bandage but do not remove the dressing.

5 If the bleeding continues, put another dressing on top and wrap another firm bandage around it. Keep applying pressure with your hands around the wound.

6 If the child is pale or drowsy, the child may be in shock. Lie the child down, and raise the legs on a folded blanket or pillow. Keep the child warm with a blanket or coat, being careful not to overheat. If the child is thirsty, wet the lips with a wet facewasher or cloth. Do not give any food or water. For more information see **Shock** (p. 55).

7 Gently place the amputated part in a clean plastic bag, and seal the bag.

8 Place the sealed bag in a container filled with water and a few ice cubes. Do not let the body part come in direct with the ice, as it can cause damage.

9 Keep reassuring the child until the ambulance arrives.

Bleeding from the ear
See **Head injuries** (p. 95).

What to do

1 Place the child in a comfortable position, for example on the injured side with the head tilted downwards. This will allow blood and fluid to drain freely.

2 Cover the ear with a clean dressing or cloth, and keep it in place with a loose bandage or adhesive tape.

3 Call an ambulance.

Finger jam injuries

Minor or serious injuries to a child's fingers and hands can result if they are jammed in a fast-closing, heavy house or building door, car door, or the wheel of an exercise bike.

Minor injury
What to do

1   If the child's finger is not bleeding and appears bruised only, make an ice-pack by wrapping ice or frozen peas in a damp cloth. Wrap this around the finger to help reduce the pain and swelling.

2   If the finger is painful, looks deformed or is difficult to move, take the child to a hospital or a doctor, as the finger may be dislocated or broken. See **Fractured or Dislocated Finger (p. 68)**.

Major injury
What to do

If a finger is amputated, do not panic. Most amputated parts can be successfully reattached. If the wound is serious and bleeding, treat as for a major wound (see pp. 54–5).

1   Calm and reassure the child.

2   Apply firm pressure to the wound using a sterile dressing, clean cloth or towel.

3   Hold the hand as high as possible, preferably above chest height.

4   Keep the dressing in place by wrapping a bandage firmly around it. Make sure it is not too tight — there should be no tingling or throbbing. If necessary, loosen the bandage, but do not remove the dressing.

5   If the bleeding continues, put another dressing on top, and wrap another firm bandage around it. Apply pressure with your hands around the wound. Keep doing this until the bleeding stops.

6   Call an ambulance.

7   If a finger or fingertip is amputated, gently place the amputated part in a clean plastic bag, and seal the bag.

8   Place the sealed bag in a container filled with water and a few ice cubes. Do not let the body part come in direct contact with the ice, as it can cause damage.

9   Keep reassuring the child until the ambulance arrives.

Nose bleed

Nose bleeds are common in children, particularly on hot days or during exercise. While a nose bleed may look serious, it is easily controlled.

What to do

1   Ask the child to sit with the head slightly forward.

2   Put a cool wet cloth over the bridge of the nose.

3   Pinch the soft part of the child's nose for at least 10 minutes, or until the bleeding has stopped. Older children can do this for themselves. If the child has been exercising, it may take 20 minutes or longer for the bleeding to stop.

4   Encourage the child to avoid blowing the nose for a few hours.

Bleeding from the mouth
See **Teeth injuries** (p. 112).

Bone, muscle and joint injuries

Facts

Injuries to bones, muscles and joints often happen when children are playing. Falls from playground equipment, bicycles, skateboards, rollerblades (in-line skates), trampolines, furniture, and during sport can result in fractures, dislocations, sprains, strains, cuts and bruises.

Children have weak bones compared to those of adults, and these can easily break as the result of a fall or other injury. Less common in young children are dislocations, sprains and strains.

At the end of a long bone, such as in an arm or leg, children up to about 16 years have what is called a growth plate or 'zone of growth'. This area is weaker than the bone or ligament, and injuries to the growth plate are common.

Young children are at risk of injury to the area surrounding their elbows as a result of being lifted or swung around by their wrists — this is known as a 'pulled elbow'.

For many children sport provides fun, fitness, friendship, increased self-esteem and skills. All too often, however, children are injured. Those aged 10–14 years who play competitive sports, particularly contact sports, commonly experience fractures and dislocations.

Competitive sports that commonly result in injuries are Australian Rules football, rugby, soccer, cricket, basketball and netball.

Spinal injuries in children are rare. The most likely causes are falls and car accidents. In addition to fractures, spinal injuries can result from a fall from a trampoline or climbing equipment. Older children, particularly teenagers, sometimes receive spinal injuries during water sports or as a result of diving into shallow water.

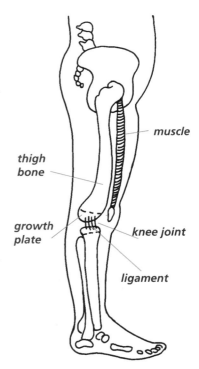

muscle

thigh bone

growth plate

knee joint

ligament

Prevention

Safe nursery furniture

Young toddlers frequently fall from nursery furniture such as high chairs, cots, prams, strollers and baby walkers. For prevention strategies see **Head injuries** (pp. 92–4).

Sports safety

Sporting injuries are more likely to happen if muscles are tight, sprains and strains have not healed before participating in further sport, or if a child is generally unfit.

A child should never be forced to play a particular sport. Emphasising 'winning at any cost' can also place a child under too much pressure, and increase the chance of injury. All children should be encouraged to participate in a sport of their choice, simply for enjoyment.

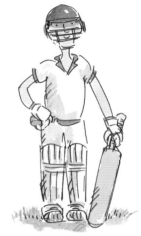

- Warm-up and cool-down exercises to increase flexibility are essential before and after playing sport or exercising.
- Many sports have modified rules, playing fields and equipment for children, and use qualified coaches who place an emphasis on safe training methods and play, and who are qualified in first aid.
- Insist that a child wear safety equipment appropriate to the sport; for example, mouthguards and face shields, helmets, footwear, knee pads, shin guards and gloves. When a child is playing outdoors, a hat and sunscreen are essential.
- Children should be matched for size, ability and maturity, rather than age. Delay heavy contact sports until after puberty.
- Don't allow a child who is feeling tired or unwell to play sport.
- When rollerblading (in-line skating) or skateboarding, a child should wear a bicycle helmet in addition to wrist, chin, elbow and knee protectors. Good footwear is required when skateboarding. Do not allow your child to wear thongs or sandals, or to skate in bare feet. Skating on roads should be forbidden.

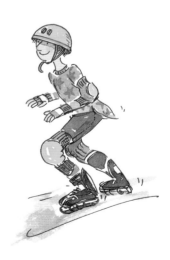

- Trampolines are popular, but are not recommended for children under 6 years. Older children need to be closely supervised to make sure that only one child at a time uses the trampoline, and attempts only simple jumps.
- A trampoline must be placed well clear of other obstacles on a soft undersurface such as grass, tan bark or sand. Check the trampoline regularly for signs of wear and tear, and place safety pads over the steel frame and springs.
- In addition to learning to swim, children must be taught to always check the depth of water before diving, particularly if the water is murky or unclear.
- Never lift a child, or swing the child around, by the wrists.

  See also **Traffic accidents** (pp. 113–15).

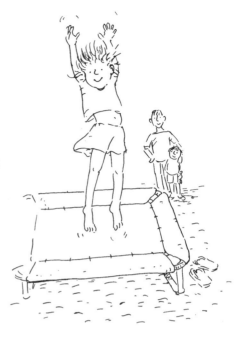

First aid

Sprains, strains and bruises (soft-tissue injuries)

Sprains, strains and bruises involve soft tissues such as ligaments, muscles and blood vessels. Sometimes it is hard to tell the difference between a bad sprain or strain and a fracture. If you are not sure, always treat it as a fracture. See **Fractures** (pp. 64–70).

While the symptoms differ, the first aid is the same for all.

Sprains

Ligaments hold bones together at a joint. They can sometimes be stretched or torn, resulting in a sprain.

What to look for
➤ pain around the joint
➤ swelling
➤ reduced movement
➤ bruising.

Strains

Muscles are attached to bones, and allow the body to move. Muscles can become over-stretched and sometimes torn, resulting in a strain.

What to look for
➤ sudden sharp pain
➤ limb weakness
➤ stiffness and cramping.

Bruises

Bruises are common in children. They occur when the tiny blood vessels under the skin are damaged. Blood moves into the soft tissues, causing the area to swell and change colour.

What to look for
➤ pain
➤ tenderness
➤ change in colour of the skin (red, purple or black)
➤ swelling.

What to do

1 *Help the child to support and rest the injured part in the most comfortable position. If it is a leg or arm, prop it up with a pillow or folded blanket.*

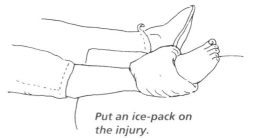

Put an ice-pack on the injury.

2 *Make an ice-pack by wrapping ice or frozen peas in a damp cloth. Do not put ice directly on the skin, as it can cause damage.*
   Put the ice-pack on the injury for 10–20 minutes:
   (a) every 2 hours for the first 24 hours,
   (b) every 4 hours for a further 24 hours.

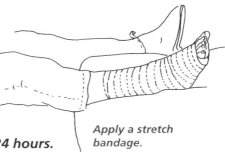

Apply a stretch bandage.

3 *After each ice-pack treatment, wrap a crepe or stretch bandage firmly over the injury and surrounding area.*

4 *Do not apply any heat in the first 48 hours, as this will make the injury worse.*

63

5 *If the injury doesn't improve, take the child to a doctor.*

Dislocation

A dislocation happens when one or more bones are forced apart at a joint. It may also involve a fracture.

What to look for
➤ severe pain
➤ loss of movement
➤ limb looks deformed
➤ swelling and bruising.

What to do

1 *Do not try to put the bone back into the joint. This can cause more damage and increase pain.*

2 *Help the child to support the injured part in the most comfortable position. If it is a leg or arm, prop it up with a pillow, or folded blanket or clothing.*

3 *Make an ice-pack by wrapping ice or frozen peas in a damp cloth. Do not put ice directly on the skin, as it can cause damage. Put the ice-pack on the injured area.*

4 *Call an ambulance.*

Fractures

Children's bones are more likely to bend and crack than to break completely. These are known as greenstick fractures. Sometimes the bone may break through the skin (an open fracture), or the fracture can damage nerves or organs.

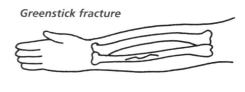
Greenstick fracture

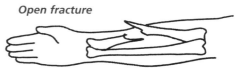
Open fracture

A growth-plate injury may be minor or severe. If minor, it may look like a sprain (see **Sprains, strains and bruises**, pp. 62–3). If severe, it may look like a fracture or even a dislocation. If not treated properly, the injury can result in joint deformity.

Sometimes it is hard to tell whether a child has a fracture, a dislocation or a serious sprain. If you are not sure what the injury is, treat it as a fracture.

What to look for
➤ may hear the snap of the bone
➤ pain made worse by trying to move
➤ the limb does not move normally
➤ the limb may look deformed
➤ a grating sound if the limb is moved
➤ tenderness over the bone
➤ swelling, and possibly bruising.

What to do

1   *Calm and reassure the child.*

2   *Stop any bleeding, and cover any wound with a clean cloth or sterile dressing.*

3   *Broken bones can bleed heavily, and this can be made worse if the child moves. If in a safe area, do not move the child. Do not try to straighten the limb. Help support the injured part in a comfortable position to reduce any pain by propping it up with a pillow or blanket or folded clothing.*

4   *All painful and severe fractures should be transported by ambulance to hospital. Ambulance officers and paramedics will treat the fracture and pain.*

5   *If you are a long way from ambulance help, you may need to support and keep the injured part still by using a sling or splint, as follows. If bandages aren't available, make use of common household materials; for example, make a sling using clothing (such as a jumper, tie or belt). You can also make a splint from a rolled-up newspaper, magazine or towel, or with a stick. If you do use a sling or splint, check with the child that it isn't too tight, that there isn't any throbbing or tingling, and loosen the sling or splint if necessary.*

Slings and splints

Fractured collar bone

What to do

1   *Calm and reassure the child.*

2   *Bend the arm on the injured side, with the fingers pointing to the opposite shoulder.*

3 Put an open triangular bandage over the arm with its point at the bent elbow.

4 Gently fold the bandage under the bent arm, and bring the bottom of the bandage around the child's back to the opposite shoulder.

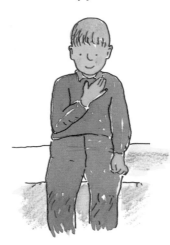
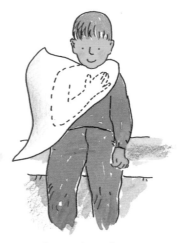
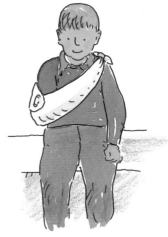

Bend the injured arm.　　Put a triangular bandage over the arm.　　Fold and tie the bandage.

5 Adjust the height of the sling, and then tie the ends near the collar bone on the uninjured side.

6 Tuck in the point between the bandage and the lower arm. Keep it in place with a safety pin.

7 Take the child to a doctor, or if the injury is painful and severe call an ambulance.

Fractured upper arm

What to do

1 Calm and reassure the child.

2 If the injury is close to the elbow, see **Fractured Elbow** (p. 67). Otherwise, make a sling as follows.

3 Make two loops in a narrow bandage. If a bandage is unavailable, use a tie or belt.

4 Bring the loops together, and put them over the wrist of the injured arm.

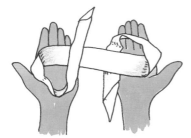

Tie two loops in a narrow bandage, and bring them together.

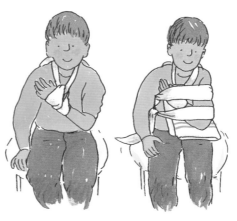

Tie the bandage around the neck.

Pad, and tie the arm to the chest.

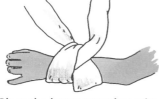

Place the loops over the wrist.

5   Gently bend the injured arm towards the opposite shoulder, and tie the two ends of the bandage around the neck.

6   Place some padding between the injured arm and the chest. Tie two broad bandages around the injured arm and the chest, above and below the fracture.

7   Take the child to a doctor, or if the injury is painful and severe call an ambulance.

Fractured elbow, or fractured upper arm near the elbow

What to do

1   Calm and reassure the child.

2   Don't try to bend the elbow. Lie the child down, and pad between the injured arm and the body.

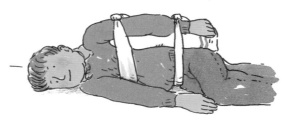

Pad, and tie the arm to the body.

3   Tie the injured arm to the body using two broad bandages, one above and one below the elbow.

4   Take the child to a doctor, or if the injury is painful or severe call an ambulance.

67

Fractured lower arm or wrist

What to do

1 *Calm and reassure the child.*

2 *Place a rolled-up newspaper, magazine or towel along the injured arm from the elbow to the middle of the child's fingers. Tie it in place at both ends of the lower arm, but not over the injury.*

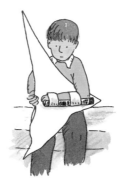
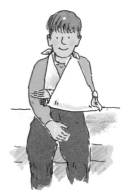

Make a splint, and tie with broad bandages.

Tie a triangular bandage around the neck.

3 *Place a triangular bandage over the child's shoulder and chest, with the point towards the elbow on the injured side.*

4 *Place the injured arm across the chest, with the hand slightly higher than the elbow. Bring the lower end of the bandage up to the shoulder on the injured side. Tie the two ends together above the collar bone.*

5 *Fold the point forward, and keep it in place with a safety pin.*

6 *Take the child to a doctor, or if the injury is painful and severe call an ambulance.*

Fractured or dislocated finger

What to do

1 *Calm and reassure the child.*

2 *Do not try to put the bones back into place, as this can sometimes make the injury worse.*

3 *If possible, make a splint using a small object such as an icecream stick; tie the fingers together with a bandage.*

4 *Place the child's arm in a sling to help reduce the swelling. See Fractured collar bone (pp. 65–6).*

5 *Take the child to a hospital or a doctor.*

Fractured leg or hip

What to do

1 *Calm and reassure the child.*

2 *Pad between the legs, using a blanket or towel, and then gently move the uninjured leg next to the injured one.*

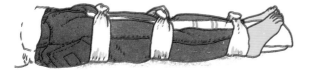

Pad between the legs, and tie together with broad bandages.

3 *Slide three broad bandages under the ankles, knees and thighs. Tie them together on the uninjured side.*

4 *Call an ambulance.*

Fractured kneecap

What to do
Do not change the position of the knee or try to straighten the leg, as this can cause more damage.

1 *Calm and reassure the child.*

2 *Put plenty of padding under the injured knee. Use a towel, jumper or folded blanket.*

3 *Call an ambulance.*

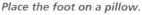

Place the foot on a pillow.

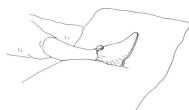

Fractured foot or ankle

What to do
Do not remove the child's shoe and sock unless severe swelling or pain makes it necessary.

1 *Calm and reassure the child.*

Fold the pillow, and tie.

2 *Wrap the injured foot in a pillow or folded blanket, and hold it together using three narrow bandages.*

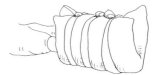

69

3 *Raise the foot slightly.*

4 *Call an ambulance.*

Neck and spinal injuries

The spinal cord sends messages to and from the brain to all parts of the body. It is protected by the spinal column, a series of small bones called vertebrae; these are supported by strong ligaments and muscles. Sometimes the spinal column can be fractured without damaging the spinal cord; however, if it is damaged, it can't be repaired. Damage to the spinal cord may cause permanent loss of movement and feeling in all areas below the injury.

What to look for
➤ back or neck pain
➤ loss of strength or control of arms or legs
➤ loss of feeling, numbness or tingling.

What to do
You may not be able to tell if a child has a spinal injury. If the child has been in a car accident or hit by a car for example, treat as if the child may have a spinal injury.

1 *Unless the child is unconscious or in an unsafe area, do not move the child, as this may damage the spinal cord. If you must move the child to a safe place, pull the child gently with the help of another person rather than lift, keeping the child's neck and back straight. If the child is in water, move the child only if the child is unconscious or at risk of drowning.*

2 *Ask someone to call an ambulance.*

3 *If the child becomes unconscious while you are waiting for the ambulance, follow the **Life-threatening emergencies chart** (front flap) until the ambulance arrives. Try to keep the spine straight.*

4 *If the child is conscious, be reassuring. Keep the child still and steady by holding the head with your hands. Keep the child warm with a blanket or overcoat until the ambulance arrives.*

Hold the head still.

Burns

Facts

Burns can be caused by:

- the sun
- hot liquids
- flames
- contact with a hot object
- electricity
- chemicals.

Children under 4 years of age, especially those aged between 1 and 2 years, are most likely to be burnt as a result of tipping hot tea or coffee over themselves. They also get burns from taps, kettles, kitchen appliances, heaters and stoves.

A child's sensitive skin burns more easily and deeply than an adult's. How bad a burn will be depends upon the source of heat, the time the child is exposed to it, the temperature, the size and the site of the burn. The quicker the first aid, the less likelihood there is of scarring.

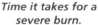

Time it takes for a severe burn.

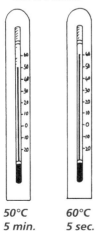

50°C
5 min.

60°C
5 sec.

Hot water burn

A severe burn will happen in 5 minutes at about 50°C, or in 5 seconds at about 60°C.

A cup of tea or coffee with milk will be at 70°C or more; a cup of tea or coffee without milk will be at 80°C or more.

Flame burn

Many house fires are started by children playing with matches and cigarette lighters, but death results more often from smoke inhalation than from burns. Flame burns from flammable liquids such as turpentine and lawnmower fuel are more common in older children, especially teenagers.

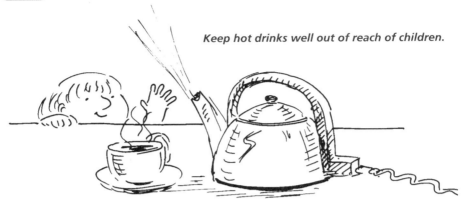

Keep hot drinks well out of reach of children.

Electrical burn

The most common type of electrical injury experienced by children is a burn. Preschoolers are at risk when playing with electrical appliances, by biting cords, placing objects in power-point sockets, or by coming into contact with faulty wiring.

Prevention

Sunburn

Regardless of skin colour, children have sensitive skin that burns easily. It is possible for a child to be burnt on overcast and cloudy or windy days.

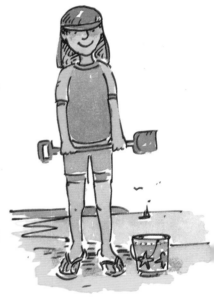

- Provide shade outdoors.
- Make sure your child wears a broadbrimmed or legionnaire-style hat and clothing that protects the body, arms and legs, as well as SPF15+ sunscreen on any exposed skin. Shade, hats and clothing are best for a young baby. Apply only small amounts of chemical-free sunscreen to the face, hands and feet.
- Buy specially designed lycra sunsuits that block out UV rays for children to wear at the beach or while playing outside.

Sunsuit.

Hot liquid burn (scald)

Young toddlers are curious, and love to copy others as they practise learning new skills. They will reach up to see what is in a cup, pull on a kettle cord or saucepan handle, turn knobs, taps and dials. The kitchen and bathroom are particularly dangerous areas.

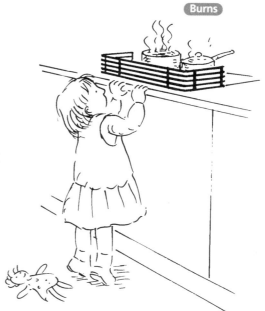

- Never leave a child alone in the kitchen or bathroom. A toddler may be safer in a playpen or a high chair for a short time while you are preparing meals. See **Safety products** (p. 15).
- Consider using door barriers in the kitchen and bathroom. You can buy them or make one yourself out of chipboard or perspex. See **Safety products** (p. 15).
- Keep hot drinks, teapots, coffee pots and kettles away from the edge of a table or bench.
- A mug is less likely to tip over than a cup and saucer. Buy insulated mugs with lids.
- Use non-slip placemats instead of a tablecloth.

Fit a stoveguard.

- Never underestimate a child's reach. Keep a long, dangling kettle cord well out of reach, or replace it with a curly cord. Consider buying a cordless kettle. See **Safety products** (p. 16).
- Empty any unused water from a kettle or saucepan after it is boiled.
- Turn all pot handles inwards, and use the back burners of the stove if possible, or fit a stove guard around the top. See **Safety products** (p. 16).
- Microwave ovens heat food to scalding temperatures very quickly. Always stir and taste before giving microwaved food or drink to a child. Place the microwave oven out of reach at the back of the bench.
- When filling the bath, put in cold water first, then add water until the bath water is warm. Check the temperature with your elbow, or use a thermometer — comfortable temperatures for babies range from 37–39°C. Never leave a child under 5 years alone in a bath. See also **Drowning** (pp. 85–8).
- Turn taps off tightly or use taps with specially designed anti-scald devices. If this isn't possible, consider taking the hot-water tap cover off each time after use so that just the spindle remains, or cut a cross in an empty plastic drink container, and fit it over the tap to make it hard for a child to turn it on.
- Set your household hot water system to 50–55°C.
- Have a plumber install a tempering valve that presets a safe maximum hot water temperature, or if you need a new hot-water system choose one that allows you some flexibility and control over the temperature.

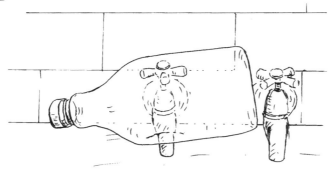

Cut a cross in a plastic bottle, and fit it over the hot tap.

Flame burn

- Lock matches, cigarette lighters, fire lighters and flammable liquids away. Keep any handbag (especially a visitor's bag) out of reach as the bag may contain a cigarette lighter or matches. See also **Poisoning** (pp. 101–2).
- Use a heater guard to prevent children from getting too close to open fires, gas space heaters, electric radiators and pot-bellied stoves.
- Choose close-fitting nightwear for children with the 'Low fire danger' or 'Styled to reduce fire danger' labels.
- Install smoke detectors; see **Safety products** (p. 16). Keep a fire blanket or fire extinguisher in the kitchen.
- Have a fire exit plan that all the family understand and practise. Teach children to crawl low in smoke, and to find two ways out of the house to a meeting place. Do not use the deadlocks on doors at night.
- Never leave children alone in a car, as they may play with the cigarette lighter.
- Keep children well away from a barbecue or open fire, even when not in use, as they may still contain hot coals or ash.

Use a fireguard.

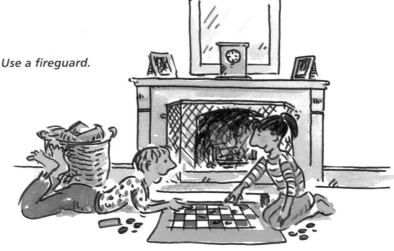

Smoke detectors

There are two types to choose from: electric with battery back-up, and battery operated. Replace the battery every 12 months.

Electrical burn

Cords, switches and electrical equipment fascinate children.

- Place a playpen around your stereo or video unit.
- Switch off electrical appliances at the power point, and unplug them after use. Make sure all cords are out of reach.
- Use a powerboard instead of double adaptors or extension cords. Use portable safety switches with power tools.
- Replace frayed electrical cords.
- Store the hairdryer and electric shaver in a locked cupboard in the bathroom. Do not use them if a child is having a bath. Avoid using an electric heater on the floor.
- Keep a hot iron and its cord out of reach of a child. Consider placing a playpen around the ironing board. See **Safety products** (p. 15).
- Safety switches (residual current devices) cut off power in a fraction of a second if there's a fault or an interruption to the normal flow of electricity. Different types give whole-house protection, and are fitted to the main switchboard, or give partial-house protection, such as those fitted to individual power points and circuits. Seek advice from a qualified electrician as to the best option to suit your situation.
- Use power-point covers in low-lying sockets. Use them even if you have a safety switch. See **Safety products** (p. 16).
- Do not use an electric blanket or a hot water bottle on a child's bed.

Chemical burn

- Store all chemicals and cleaning products in locked cupboards in the house, garage and gardening shed. See **Safety products** (p. 15).
- Dishwasher detergent can burn a child's skin and throat. Buy it in a plastic container with a child-resistant cap, and lock it away. Keep the door of the dishwasher closed at all times.
- When buying a dishwasher, choose one with a child-resistant catch. See also **Poisoning** (pp.101–2).

First aid

Sunburn

What to do

1   *Place a cool, wet towel or cloth on the burnt area. Do not use ice, as this can stick to the skin.*

2   *Give the child some water to drink.*

3   *If the burnt area starts to blister, take the child to a doctor.*

Flame and hot liquid burn

What to do

1   *If the child's clothing is on fire, push the child to the ground. Smother the flames by rolling the child over several times, or wrap a woollen blanket or fire blanket around the child.*

Cool a burn with water.

2   *Calm and reassure the child.*

3   *Immediately cool the burnt or scalded area with cold water for at least 10 minutes. This is important to reduce the severity of the burn. Do not use ice, as this can stick to the skin.*

4   *Remove any clothing that has been burnt, or soaked by boiling water. Do not pull the clothes over the child's head, cut them off instead. If clothing is stuck to the skin, leave it or cut around it. Remove any shoes or jewellery in case the area starts to swell.*

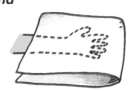

5   *Do not break any blisters, or apply creams, ointments or butter to the burn. Cover the burn with a clean, non-fluffy dressing or cloth, such as a clean sheet or pillow case.*

Wrap the burn in a clean cloth.

6   *All burns larger than a 20c coin should be seen by a doctor. If a burn is very painful, covers a large area of skin, is pale, waxy or charred, call an ambulance.*

7 *If the child becomes drowsy or pale, lie the child down, and raise the legs using a pillow or folded blanket, and call an ambulance. See **Shock** (p. 55). If the child becomes unconscious while you are waiting, follow the **Life-threatening emergencies chart** (front flap) until the ambulance arrives.*

Chemical burn

What to do

Chemical swallowed

1 *If the child has swallowed a chemical that burns or is caustic, such as dishwasher detergent, drain or oven cleaner, give the child sips of milk or water. Do not force the child to drink.*

2 *Take the substance and the child to the phone. Call the Poisons Information Centre (☎ 13 11 26) immediately, anywhere in Australia, 24 hours a day, and follow their instructions. Do not make the child vomit.*

Chemical on skin

1 *If the chemical is on the skin, remove any clothing that has come in contact with it, and wash the skin with plenty of cold water for 15–20 minutes.*

2 *Call an ambulance.*

Electrical burn

What to do

1 *Avoid touching the child if the child is in contact with an electrical appliance or wire — you risk electrocution. Switch off the power to the appliance or at the main fuse box.*

2 *If the child is unconscious, follow the **Life-threatening emergencies chart** (front flap), and call an ambulance.*
   If the child is conscious, look for any burns. There will usually be two burns, one burn where the electricity entered, and another where it left the child's body. Call an ambulance. While you are waiting, cool the burnt areas with cold water for at least 10 minutes.

Choking, suffocation and strangulation

Facts

The thought of their child choking is often the parents' worst fear. It is, however, rarely life-threatening. In most cases your child will be able to cough up any blockage without help.

Young children do not have a full set of teeth, which makes chewing food difficult, and they have very narrow airways. Foods such as apple, raw carrot, celery, popcorn, meat and peanuts are not easily chewed and swallowed. Of all these foods, peanuts generally cause more children to choke. A running, laughing or crying child is more likely to choke on food.

Young children often put things in their mouths. Small objects that fit into a cylinder about the size of a film canister can cause a child under 3 years to choke. Some of these objects include coins, small toys, pen tops, nails and screws, buttons, disc batteries, pebbles.

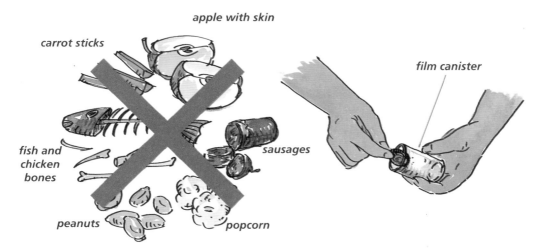

apple with skin

carrot sticks

film canister

fish and chicken bones

sausages

peanuts

popcorn

Young children may choke on these foods.   **Small objects may cause a child to choke.**

78

Babies and young children are at risk of suffocation and strangulation in unsafe sleeping situations. This includes:

- sleeping with adults
- sleeping on a water bed, couch, beanbag, or sheepskin rug
- getting wedged in a gap between a mattress and the cot sides
- sleeping face down
- sleeping in nightwear with a cord or ribbon around the neck
- sleeping in a cot that has a string or cord attached (for example, a balloon with a string), or in a cot that is near blind cords.

Prevention

Choking

Many foods are light, and easily inhaled by children. Others are hard to chew, and get caught in the airway.

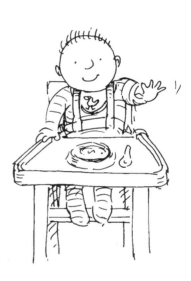

- Encourage your child to sit quietly when eating and drinking.
- Do not give nuts, particularly peanuts, and popcorn to a child under 5 years. A thin layer of peanut butter or hazelnut spread on bread is a good alternative.
- Children under 3 years are most at risk of choking on carrot sticks, pieces of apple, meat, fish and chicken bones. Apples and carrots should be grated or cooked. Fruits such as ripe pears, bananas, peaches or apricots are softer and safer to eat.
- Remove sharp or small bits of bone from fish, chicken and meat, or use boneless fillets. Cut all food into small pieces.
- Cut sausages and frankfurts lengthways, and then into small pieces.
- Never leave your baby alone with a propped-up bottle.

Young children, particularly those under 3 years, often put objects in their mouths. Toys with small parts, and small objects lying around on the floor or within easy reach, can become a problem.

- Keep small objects such as safety pins, buttons, coins, small disc batteries, nails, screws, polystyrene beads and pen tops out of reach.
- Choose toys suitable for your child's age by reading the advice label on the toy packaging.
- Do not give uninflated balloons to young children.

Suffocation

Making the right — and safe — choice in nursery furniture helps both you and your child to sleep peacefully.

- A cot mattress must be firm and fit snugly. The spaces between cot bars should be between 50 mm and 85 mm; the depth of the cot must be a minimum of 500 mm from the top of the mattress to the top of the cot. Secondhand and old cots can be dangerous if they don't meet nursery furniture safety standards. Contact the Federal Bureau of Consumer Affairs, Department of Business and Fair Trading (Victoria) or the child safety organisation in your state or territory for further information.

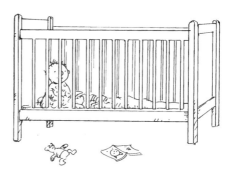

Choose nursery furniture that meets the Australian Standard.

- Before use, remove any plastic cover on a cot or bassinet mattress.
- Sheepskin rugs, if used, should have a short pile and be covered by a sheet.
- Pillows are not necessary for children under 2 years.
- A baby shouldn't sleep or be left alone on a water bed. If the baby rolls over, the face may sink into the bed.
- Tie a knot in discarded plastic bags, used plastic wrap and dry-cleaning bags, and keep them out of reach of toddlers.
- A child's toy box should have air holes and a slow-closing hinge.
- Take the door off a refrigerator if it is no longer in use and left sitting in the backyard or awaiting hard rubbish collection.

Strangulation

- Place the cot or child's bed well away from curtains or blinds with long cords. Cut or tie the cords so that they are out of reach of a toddler — consider attaching a tie-down device on the wall or window frame, or attach a rod ('wand') to a blind in place of a cord.
- Do not tie balloons or toys with long strings to the cot.
- Do not allow your young child to play unsupervised with a rope, cord or belt.
- Your baby shouldn't sleep in clothing that is loose, has a hood, or a cord or ribbon around the neck. Remove the feeding bib before putting the child down to sleep.
- Never leave your baby alone while the baby is asleep in a baby bouncer or car restraint with loose straps.

First aid

Choking
A choking child may have a partial or complete blockage of the airway.

Partial blockage
The child can breathe, speak, cry or cough.

What to do

1   *Reassure the child. Encourage the child to keep coughing to remove the foreign material. Don't try to remove it, as this may totally block the airway.*

2   *Place the baby or child over your lap, with the head in a downward position. This will help the coughing child clear the blockage. If the child turns blue, becomes limp or unconscious or can't clear the blockage in a few minutes, call an ambulance. See **Total blockage** below.*

Total blockage
The child cannot breathe, speak, cry or cough.

What to do
Baby or small child

1   *Call an ambulance.*

2   *Place the baby or child over your lap, with the child's head in a downward position.*

3   *Give up to four firm back blows between the shoulder blades, using the lower part (heel) of your hand, to try to dislodge the foreign material.*

4   *If the child is still not breathing, place your hands on either side of the child's chest under the armpits. Give up to four quick squeezing thrusts, using both hands simultaneously.*

5   *If the child is still not breathing, follow the **Life-threatening emergencies chart** (front flap), while waiting for the ambulance to arrive.*
    Because of the blockage, there may be some initial resistance felt when attempting mouth-to-mouth resuscitation.

6 **Keep repeating the chest thrusts as above, every minute, alternating with resuscitation, until the ambulance arrives.**

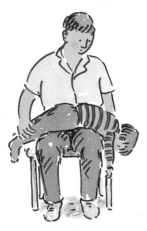
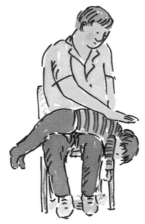
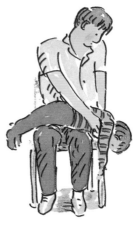

Place a baby or small child across your knees.

For a baby or small child, give firm back blows.

For a baby or small child, give chest thrusts.

Large child

1 **Call an ambulance.**

2 **Place the child on one side, with the head low.**

3 **Give up to four firm back blows between the shoulder blades, using the lower part (heel) of your hand, to try to dislodge the object.**

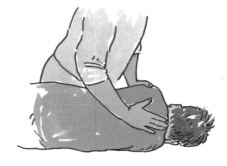

For an older child, give firm back blows.

4 **If the child is still not breathing, place one hand against the armpit and place the other next to it. Give four downward thrusts, keeping your hand on the chest at all times.**

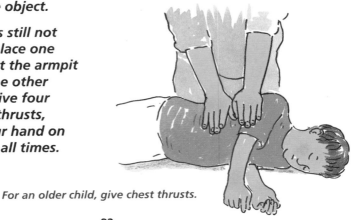

For an older child, give chest thrusts.

82

5 *If the child is still not breathing, follow the **Life-threatening emergencies chart** (front flap), until the ambulance arrives.*
Because of the blockage, there may be some initial resistance felt when attempting mouth-to-mouth resuscitation.

6 *Keep repeating the chest thrusts as above, every minute, alternating with resuscitation, until the ambulance arrives.*

Swallowed object

What to do

1 *If you think a child has swallowed an object, call the Poisons Information Centre (☎ 13 11 26) for advice, anywhere in Australia, 24 hours a day, or consult a doctor.*

Suffocation and strangulation

What to do

1 *If you can, remove whatever has caused the child to have difficulty breathing.*

2 *If the child is unconscious, call an ambulance, and follow the **Life-threatening emergencies chart** (front flap) until the ambulance arrives.*

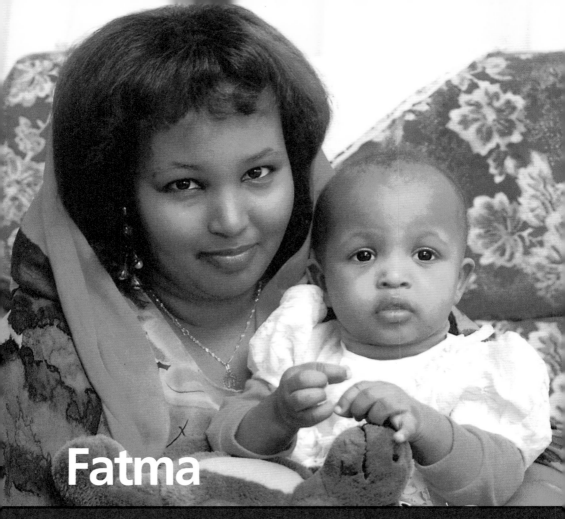

Fatma

Fatma's first birthday party was not quite the celebration her mum and dad had planned. A small piece of plastic from a toy she was given as a gift caused her to choke.

'It's something I would never want to go through again', said her mum, Amina. 'One minute Fatma was happily playing, the next she was coughing and spluttering. She couldn't cry, and she started to turn blue and gasp for air. I didn't know what to do!'

Fortunately her uncle who was at the party did — he grabbed Fatma, and placed her over his knees and gave her firm blows on the back. Out popped the toy, and she started to breathe again. In the meantime Amina called for an ambulance.

By the time it arrived, Fatma was back to normal and happily playing again.

'We will always be grateful to our brother who saved Fatma's life. It made me realise how important it is to know first aid. Next time I'll be

Drowning

Facts

Drowning is the most common cause of death of children under 5 years of age. Those most at risk are aged 1–3 years. Half the drownings are in backyard swimming pools; the remainder are in baths, spas, wading pools, buckets, dams, rivers and creeks.

A toddler can easily overbalance, as the head and shoulders are large compared to the rest of the body. A child falling into water will have difficulty lifting the head to breathe.

A child can drown silently in a few minutes in water only a few centimetres deep. When the child loses consciousness, a large amount of water is swallowed, and vomiting is common. Death from drowning occurs due to a lack of oxygen to the brain and heart.

A child's survival depends upon early rescue and effective resuscitation.

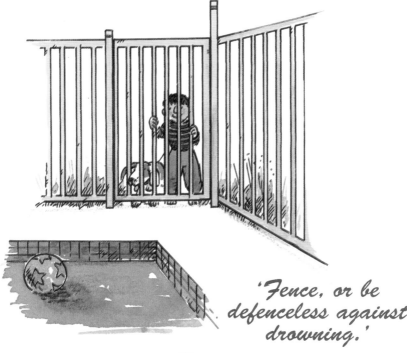

'Fence, or be defenceless against drowning.'

Prevention

Young children are curious and fearless, and are drawn to water.

- Supervision is essential at all times when a child is near or playing in water.
- Backyard pools and spas should be fenced on all sides. The fence should be Standards Australia approved, with a self-locking, self-closing gate, and maintained in good working order.
- Store away outdoor furniture or ladders, which the child could use to climb the fence.
- Empty paddling pools immediately after each use.
- Place and secure wire netting over a fish pond.
- Do not leave any children under 5 years of age unsupervised in a bath.

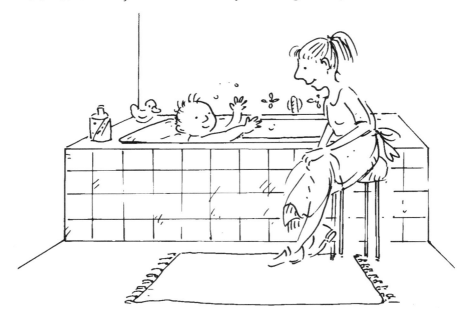

- Choose a nappy bucket with a firm fitting lid, and place it up high or in the laundry trough.
- If there is a dam on your property, provide a fenced area near the house for children to play.
- Young children cannot be 'drown proofed'. Swimming lessons are recommended from about 3 years of age, as children are better able to learn how to swim from that age. They need a lot of instruction and practice to become competent swimmers, and close supervision is still necessary.

First aid

What to do

1 *Rescue the child from the water. Use a flotation aid, if available. Get help if it isn't safe for you to do so or you cannot swim.*

2 *If the child is unconscious, start resuscitation immediately, following the **Life-threatening emergencies chart** (front flap). Do not delay or wait for help — call for help, and an ambulance. Always attempt resuscitation, even after the child has been a long time in the water. The cold water may protect the child's brain from the effects of lack of oxygen.*

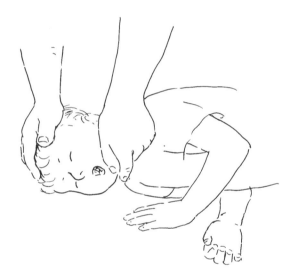

3 *If the child vomits during resuscitation, place the child on one side to clear the airway. Once it is clear, start resuscitation again.*
The child's stomach may be swollen. Do not push on it, as this increases the chances of vomiting.

4 *Continue resuscitation until the ambulance arrives.*

5 *Make sure the child is assessed in a hospital, even if the child recovers or seems all right, as lung problems may occur later.*

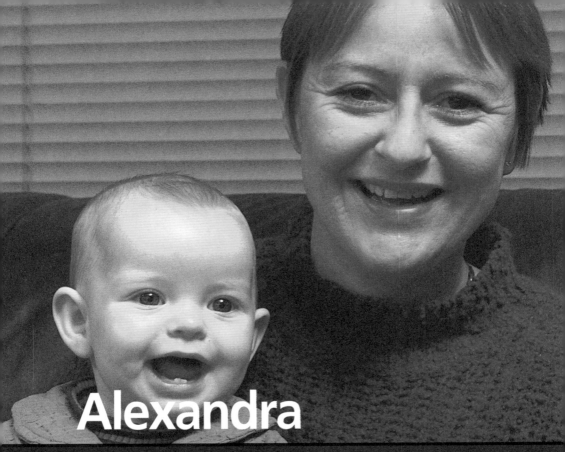

Alexandra

It is a day Chris tries to forget. But late every Wednesday afternoon she remembers how close her 9½-month-old daughter Alexandra came to drowning in a bucket. It happened in an instant, it always does. What was to be a quick wash before putting Alexandra into her pyjamas for bed, turned unexpectedly into a fight for her survival.

Chris took a bucket into the loungeroom, and added just enough warm water to sponge down Alexandra and her 3-year-old brother. In leaving her young baby for less than a minute to heat up some more water, there was enough time for Alexandra to crawl across the full length of the room. Pulling herself up to look into the bucket, she fell into it, head-first.

By the time Chris returned, Alexandra was not breathing. She had drowned in just 10 cm of water.

Chris recalls grabbing her baby, and rushing to the phone. She dialled 000, and was put through to an ambulance officer who calmly instructed her in CPR. Having recently completed a first aid and resuscitation course, Chris was able to quickly recall the procedure.

When the ambulance arrived, Chris had successfully managed to revive Alexandra.

Her message is simple: 'Always be one step ahead; never underestimate

Eye injuries

Facts

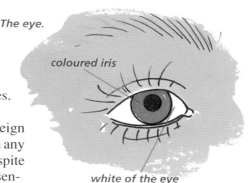

The eye.

coloured iris

white of the eye

Sight is one of our most precious senses. The body protects our eyes in bony sockets, produces tears to flush out foreign bodies, and the eyelids snap shut when any object comes too close to the face. Despite these defences, however, the eyes are sensitive and easily damaged.

Eye injuries commonly result when children play rough games or throw rocks, sticks and glass bottles. Some toys and sharp objects, such as knives, pens and scissors, are unsafe in the hands of a small child, as they may cause an eye injury if the child falls while playing. Cleaning products, ointments, cosmetics and cigarettes will also result in burns if young children rub them into their eyes.

Older children sometimes receive eye injuries when playing ball sports such as squash, tennis, badminton, cricket and Australian Rules football.

Cuts, abrasions, bruising, inflammation, or piercing of the eye can result in temporary or permanent vision loss.

Prevention

- Provide plastic eating utensils for young children.
- Keep sharp knives, bottles, jars and scissors out of the reach of toddlers.
- Read warning labels on toy packaging. Avoid buying toys that have missiles or projectiles.
- Children must understand that throwing objects when they get angry can cause others to be hurt.
- Protective eyewear should be worn if children play such sports as hockey, baseball, squash or cricket.

Sunglasses for children
Eyes are sensitive to the harmful effects of the sun, and need protection. A child is never too young to wear sunglasses. Your child can start using them

at any age, the challenge will be to keep them on! Look for the Standards Australia sticker (AS 1067), as this tells you that the sunglasses provide good protection for your child's eyes. In addition to sunglasses, a legionnaire-type hat with a brim helps to cut down the glare.

First aid

Small and loose objects

What to look for
- child rubbing eyes
- red and watering eye
- painful eye
- difficulty in opening eye.

What to do

1 *Sit the child down, calm and reassure the child, and discourage any rubbing of the eye.*

2 *Ask the child to look up, and gently pull the lower eyelid down and out.*

3 *If you can see the object on the white part of the eye, remove it by using the corner of a clean, wet piece of cloth. Do not attempt to remove an object from the coloured part of the eye.*

4 *If this doesn't work, wash out the object using cool running water from a tap or jug.*

5 *If the object cannot be removed, take the child to a doctor or a hospital emergency department.*

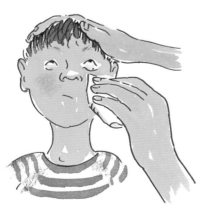
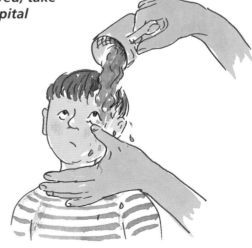

Object stuck in the eye

What to do

1 *Do not try to remove the object. Calm and lie the child down.*

2 *Cover the eye, if you can do so without putting any pressure on the eye or eyelids.*

3 *Call an ambulance.*

Wound

What to do

1 *Calm and lie the child down.*

2 *Put an eye pad or a clean cloth over the injured eye if there is bleeding.*

3 *Call an ambulance.*

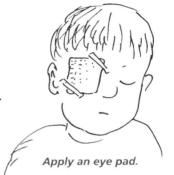

Apply an eye pad.

Chemical burn to the eye

What to look for
➤ painful eye
➤ red and watering eye
➤ swollen eyelids
➤ difficulty in opening eye.

What to do

1 *Open the child's eyelid, and wash the chemicals from the eye's surface using cool running water from a tap or jug. Continue washing the eye for 20 minutes.*

2 *Take the substance and the child to the phone. Phone the Poisons Information Centre (☎ 13 11 26), anywhere in Australia, 24 hours a day, and follow their instructions.*

3 *If the poison is caustic or petroleum-based, such as dishwasher powder, petrol or kerosene, pour water over the affected eye, and put eye pads or a clean cloth over both eyes.*

4 *Call an ambulance.*

Head injuries

Facts

Head injuries may result in bleeding, and swelling of the brain. Following a head injury, a child may have a brief loss of consciousness, followed by confusion and a lack of memory of what happened. This is known as concussion, and should be treated as a head injury.

Head injuries are commonly caused by a blow to the head or a fall from a height. Young children are most at risk of head injury from falls — they have large and heavy heads, and fall easily. The seriousness of a fall depends upon the height a child falls from, what the child falls onto, and what the child hits when falling.

Older children and adolescents receive head injuries as a result of road accidents, particularly crossing roads and bicycling, when playing sports such as football, soccer and cricket, or in the playground. Many have been injured when horse-riding and snow-skiing.

There has been a significant decrease in the number of serious head injuries since the introduction of laws throughout Australia requiring cyclists to wear helmets.

Prevention

Babies wriggle from birth, and it is not long before they learn to roll over.

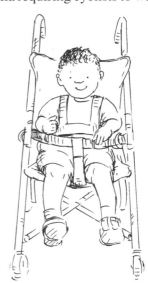

- The floor is the safest place to change a baby. If you are using a change table, choose one with a restraining strap, or always remember to keep one hand firmly on the baby.
- Use a full body harness in a pram, stroller and high chair.
- The mattress in a cot should be no thicker than 100 mm to ensure that the top of the

Use a full body harness in a pram or stroller.

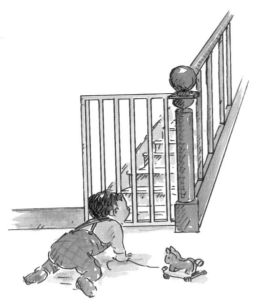

cot isn't too low. The minimum distance from the mattress to the top of the cot must be 500 mm. See also **Choking, suffocation and strangulation** (p. 80).

A child just starting to learn to walk has many minor falls. By taking the following action, serious injury can be prevented.

- Leave the cot sides down if your young child is determined to get out. Repeated attempts is a signal that it is time to consider moving the child to a low bed.
- Use stair barriers at the top and bottom of the stairs.
- Avoid babywalkers because of the high risk of injury. Many accidents are due to falls caused by tripping on mats, falling down steps, and overbalancing.
- Use rubber mats in the bath, or paint the bath with transparent non-slip paint. Many non-slip tiles and paints are available from safety flooring companies.

Once children learn to walk, they soon learn how to climb. A preschooler has the ability to reach great heights, but has no fear or understanding of the consequences of a fall.

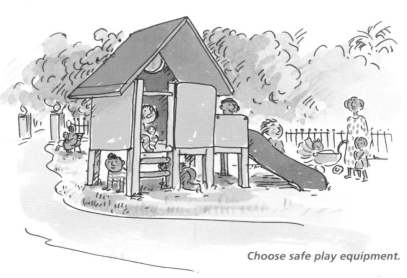

Choose safe play equipment.

- Children under 5 years of age should not be allowed to have access to heights over 1.5 metres, or older children to heights over 2 metres.
- Place tanbark or pine chips to a minimum depth of 300 mm under playground equipment. This provides a soft landing surface should a child fall.
- Bunk beds are not safe for children under 9 years of age.

As children grow and become more active, their recreational interests often expose them to higher risks of head injury.

- Bicycle helmets should be worn, even when a young child rides a tricycle in the backyard.
- In addition to wrist, elbow and knee protectors, bicycle helmets should be worn when the child is skateboarding or rollerblading (in-line skating).
- Horseriders should wear a Standards Australia approved riding helmet, and riding boots with smooth heels and soles, matched to the size of the stirrup. Horses with an even temperament and those older than 5 years are safer for young inexperienced riders.
- Children who participate in snow-skiing should wear a specially designed helmet available from some ski specialists and sports stores.

See also **Sports safety** (p. 61) and **Traffic accidents** (p. 114).

First aid

Head injuries

What to look for
➤ short period of unconsciousness
➤ confusion
➤ loss of memory
➤ nausea and/or vomiting

➤ headache
➤ paleness
➤ drowsiness
➤ pupils may be a different size.

What to do

1   *If the child is unconscious, place the child on one side. Follow the **Life-threatening emergencies chart** (front flap), and call an ambulance.*

2   *Even if the child has lost consciousness for only a short time, the child must still be assessed in hospital.*

3   *If the child has not been unconscious, watch closely for drowsiness, vomiting, or changes in behaviour. If any of these occur, take the child to a hospital.*

Bleeding from the ear
Bleeding from the ear following a blow to the head may indicate a fractured skull.

What to do

1   *Place the child in a comfortable position on the side of the injured ear with the head tilted downwards, so that blood and fluid can drain freely.*

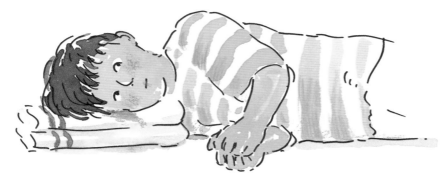

Lie the child down, on the side of the bleeding ear.

2   *Cover the ear with a clean dressing or cloth, and keep it in place with a loose bandage or adhesive tape.*

3   *Call an ambulance.*

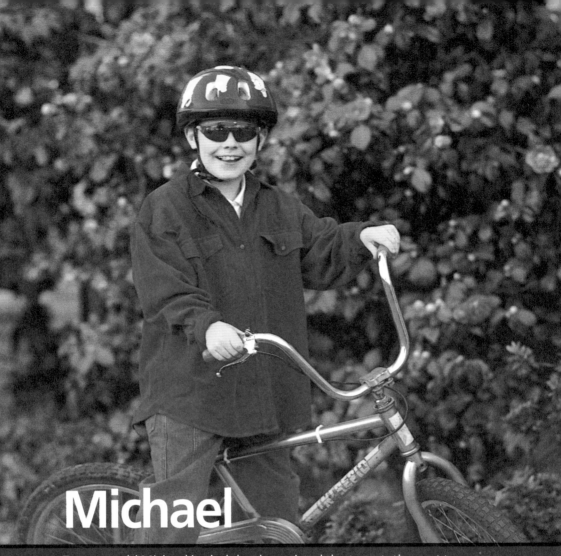

Michael

Ten-year-old Michael is glad that he resisted the temptation not to wear his bicycle helmet when going for what was to be a short ride after school with two friends. Within a few minutes of setting off from his house, his front wheel hit the kerb, and he was thrown head-first against the wind-screen of a passing car.

Fortunately for Michael, his friends and the driver of the car were able to quickly help and reassure him, and called an ambulance. He suffered mild concussion and bruising, and received five stitches in his arm. The doctor who treated him in hospital said that had Michael not been wearing a hel-met, he would undoubtedly have received severe head injuries.

Michael said that his parents had always made him and his younger sister wear helmets, even in the backyard. Sporting a bright new helmet months after the accident, Michael wants to thank his friends for their help and to let others know that wearing a helmet is a 'cool thing to do'.

Needle-stick injuries

Facts

Sometimes syringes and needles are thrown away by drug users rather than returned to a needle-exchange programme, and are found in playgrounds, gutters and laneways. The risk of a child catching HIV (the virus that causes AIDS), or some other disease such as hepatitis, after being jabbed by a needle is extremely low.

Prevention

- Children should wear closed-in footwear when playing outside or in public playgrounds.
- Young children must be taught never to pick up a needle or syringe, and if they find one to tell an adult.
- If a syringe is found in a public place, it is important to dispose of it quickly and safely to decrease the risk of anyone getting a needle-stick injury or being exposed to blood.

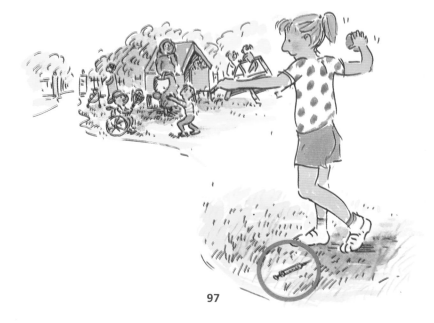

The best way to dispose of a needle and syringe is as follows:

1 *Find a screwtop, puncture-proof, plastic container, such as a fruit juice bottle or detergent container.*

2 *Place this on a flat, stable surface as close as possible to the needle and syringe.*

3 *Do not try to put the cap on the needle. Pick up the syringe by the barrel end, not the sharp end, and drop it into the container. Do not hold the container as you are placing the syringe in it. Seal it with the lid.*

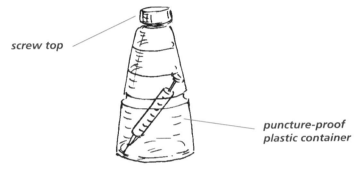

screw top

puncture-proof
plastic container

4 *Wash your hands with warm soapy water, and contact your local council's Environmental Health Officer, or a needle-exchange programme.*

First aid

What to do

1 *Immediately remove the syringe needle from the child's skin.*

2 *Gently squeeze the wound to make it bleed.*

3 *Wash the area with warm, soapy water.*

4 *Apply antiseptic as soon as possible, and cover the wound with a dressing such as a Band-Aid.*

5 *Take the child to a doctor or hospital emergency department for assessment advice and counselling.*

Poisoning

Facts

Thousands of children in Australia are poisoned each year, but fortunately there are very few deaths. Children under 4 years of age are the most likely to be poisoned, usually by swallowing a medicine, a chemical or a pesticide. Small amounts, even a teaspoon, of some poisons can be harmful. Despite what is commonly believed, children rarely die from eating poisonous plants as they taste bitter and cause intense discomfort in the mouth, causing the child to spit out the plant.

Some common household poisons

paracetamol	petrol and kerosene
tranquillisers and sedatives	bleaches, drain- and oven-cleaners
automatic dishwasher detergent	rat or mouse bait
soaps and detergents	cosmetics
cigarettes	disc batteries
mothballs	eucalyptus and tea-tree oil
alcohol	

Poisoning can also occur when a substance is inhaled, absorbed through the skin, splashed or rubbed into the eyes. The chances of inhaling a poison increases with age. Teenagers who deliberately inhale solvents from some paints, butane gas and petrol risk brain damage or death.

Prevention

Toddlers and preschoolers are active and eager to explore. They love to climb, touch and taste new things.

Some children have been known to eat or drink unusual or bad-tasting and smelling substances. Their sense of taste and smell cannot be relied upon to keep them out of danger, and they don't understand what is harmful.

All poisons should be locked away, even if they are in containers with child-resistant lids. Placing poisons up high in an unlocked cupboard is a good start, but no guarantee that your child will not climb and discover them.

The Poisons Information Centre (☎ 13 11 26), is an Australia-wide, 24-hour emergency service; it also provides information about prevention of poisoning.

Medicines (from the doctor, supermarket or chemist)

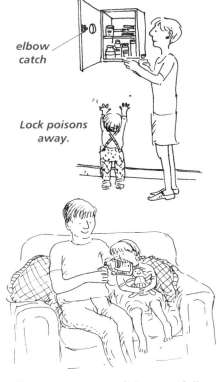

elbow catch

Lock poisons away.

- Get rid of unwanted or out-of-date medicines by returning them to the chemist. Ask for all medicines to be dispensed in a bottle with a child-resistant cap.
- Store all medicines meant for adults and children, and even those in bottles with child-resistant caps, in a poisons cabinet or cupboard with a specially designed child-resistant lock. See **Safety products** (p. 15).
- Never leave medicines or poisons on a benchtop after using or buying them. Lock them away immediately. Do not turn your back on a child when a poisonous product is within reach.
- Always measure medicine doses carefully, especially at night. Keep strictly to the number of doses allowed each day.
- Do not confuse a child by referring to medicines as lollies. Avoid taking medicines in front of children, as they tend to copy what you do.
- Use a lockable computer disk box to store medicines that need to be kept in the fridge, such as Panadol drops, insulin, some eye drops and some antibiotics.

Always measure medicines carefully.

- Keep any handbag, especially a visitor's bag, out of reach. The bag may contain medicines, cigarettes and matches, or other poisonous substances.

Cleaning products

- When buying a cleaning product, choose one in a child-resistant container, and lock it away.
- Leave chemicals in their original containers. Do not put them into empty plastic drink containers or bottles.
- Consider making your own non-toxic, all-purpose cleaner, such as a mixture of equal parts of vinegar and bicarbonate of soda.

- Dishwasher detergent can burn a child's skin and throat. Buy the detergent in a plastic bottle with a child-resistant cap, rather than in a cardboard box. Keep the door of the dishwasher closed at all times. (If you are buying a dishwater, buy one with a child-resistant catch.)
- Store medicines, chemicals, gardening products and pesticides in separate, locked cupboards.

Poisonous plants

- Learn to recognise poisonous plants, and do not plant them in your garden. If you do have poisonous plants, remove them and replace them with non-poisonous ones. See **Poisonous plants** (pp. 105–9).
- Place all poisonous indoor plants out of reach of young children, as many common indoor plants contain poisonous sap or berries. Even if the plant isn't poisonous, the dirt or potting mix may contain chemicals that will be poisonous if the child attempts to eat it.
- Teach children, particularly young children, not to touch or eat poisonous plants.
- Always supervise children in the garden.

First aid

Swallowed poison

What to look for
➤ There may be a wide range of effects or symptoms, depending upon the poison; for example, drowsiness, vomiting, stomach pain, skin irritation, paleness, breathing difficulties.
➤ The effects/symptoms may occur over hours or days.

If you think a child has eaten or drunk something poisonous, do not wait for the child to show any changes or appear unwell.

What to do

1 *If you think a child has eaten or drunk something harmful, keep calm! Very few children need instant medical treatment. You have the time to get the help you need over the phone. Remember, few poisonings are life-threatening, and rushing to the hospital or a doctor may be unnecessary. Do not rely on first aid information on packaging, as it can be out-of-date or wrong.*

2 *Do not make the child vomit. Gather up the remains of the medicine, chemical or substance, and take the container and substance and the child to the phone.*

3   *Call the Poisons Information Centre
    (☎ 13 11 26) immediately, anywhere
    in Australia, 24 hours a day, and
    follow their instructions. Don't
    hesitate to call, even if you're unsure
    that the child has taken something.*

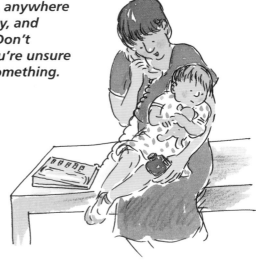

4   *If you know the poison
    is caustic, such as
    dishwasher detergent,
    drain- or oven-cleaners,
    give sips of milk or
    water, but do not force
    the child to drink. Call
    the Poisons Information
    Centre immediately,
    and follow their
    instructions.*

Call the Poisons Information Centre.

5   *If you live more than
    one hour away from
    medical help, keep a bottle of Syrup of Ipecac available. This
    will make the child vomit, **but should only be given on the
    advice of the Poisons Information Centre.***

Eating or touching a poisonous plant

What to do

1   *Stay calm. You have the time to get the help you need over
    the phone.*

2   *If you think the child has eaten some of the plant, do not
    make the child vomit. Gather some of the plant, and take it
    and the child to the phone.*

3   *Call the Poisons Information Centre (☎ 13 11 26), anywhere
    in Australia, 24 hours a day, and follow their instructions. Do
    not hesitate to call, even if you're unsure that the child has
    eaten or touched the plant.*

4   *If you live more than one hour away from medical help, keep
    a bottle of Syrup of Ipecac available. This will make the child
    vomit, **but should only be given on the advice of the
    Poisons Information Centre.***

Inhaled poison

What to do

1. *Take the child to an open window or door, or outside, to breathe in fresh air.*

2. *Take the substance and the child to the phone. Call the Poisons Information Centre (☎ 13 11 26), anywhere in Australia, 24 hours a day, and follow their instructions.*

3. *If the child becomes unconscious, follow the **Life-threatening emergencies chart** (front flap), and call an ambulance.*

Poison on the skin

What to do

1. *Remove the child's clothing if the poison has come into contact with it.*

2. *Wash the skin with plenty of cool tap water for 15–20 minutes.*

3. *Take the substance and the child to the phone. Call the Poisons Information Centre (☎ 13 11 26), anywhere in Australia, 24 hours a day, and follow their instructions.*

Poison in the eye

What to do

1. *Open the child's eyelid, and wash the substance from the eye's surface using cool running water from a tap or jug. Continue washing the eye for 20 minutes.*

2. *Take the substance and the child to the phone. Call the Poisons Information Centre (☎ 13 11 26), anywhere in Australia, 24 hours a day, and follow their instructions.*

3. *If the poison is caustic or petroleum-based, such as dishwasher powder, petrol or kerosene, wash over the affected eye using cool running water from a tap or jug.*

4. *Call an ambulance.*

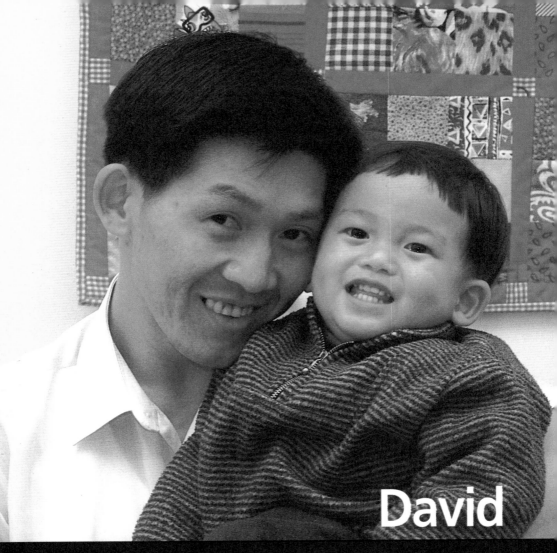

David

At 18 months of age David has discovered that not everything you swallow is good for you.

Recently he spent a day in hospital after swallowing a whole bottle of Paracetamol syrup that had been left by his bedside. David, who had a bad cold, was given a small dose of syrup in the middle of the night. His dad, Simon, was surprised to find the bottle empty the next morning.

Uncertain about what effect it could have, Simon immediately contacted the Poisons Information Centre. He is glad he did, as he was advised to get his child to hospital immediately. He later found out that large amounts of Paracetamol can be dangerous to children.

A little tired but relieved, David's parents were grateful for the advice they received. Said Simon, 'You wouldn't even know that anything had happened, David is back to his happy and active self. This should serve as a warning to other parents — lock all medicines and other poisons away.'

Poisonous plants

Do you know which plants in your garden are poisonous? Many people do not, and are often surprised by what they find. Some of the most beautiful gardens contain 'good-looking' poisonous plants. But which ones are they?

Plants with bright and colourful parts can be attractive to young children. A few can be life-threatening if eaten; others can cause skin rashes, swelling of the lips, burning of the mouth, stomach pains, vomiting and diarrhoea. Children most at risk of poisoning are under the age of 4, as they tend to experiment and put things into their mouths. Fortunately, many poisonous plants are very bitter or cause intense discomfort, especially of the lips, mouth and throat. This usually means that the plant is spat out, and so very few children die from eating poisonous plants. If a piece of the plant is eaten, it commonly causes vomiting, which naturally limits the amount of poison getting into the body.

The following table lists some commonly found poisonous plants. Many are grown in gardens, as well as indoors in domestic, or public settings. Others have become weeds and are found in waste places, laneways, paddocks or roadsides. All of these plants have resulted in children being poisoned.

The table lists each plant by its common name(s) and, as some plants have many common names, the Latin botanical name. The major identifying features are described to help you to recognise each plant.

The poisonous parts of each plant are given a toxicity rating (extreme, moderate or mild): those with an extreme rating have been known to cause death in children; those with a moderate rating can cause death but usually cause severe discomfort, requiring hospitalisation; those with a mild rating may require medical attention.

Possible symptoms are a guide to what reaction you may expect if the poisonous parts are eaten or touched. The symptoms can vary considerably, depending on the individual child's sensitivity to the poison, the amount of the plant involved, the part of the plant involved, and even the season of the year. However, most of the plants listed cause an intense stinging or burning of the skin or mouth, followed by nausea and vomiting if eaten.

There are many more poisonous plants than those mentioned here. Some are imported; others are Australian native plants. For a complete list, contact the Poisons Information Centre, your local herbarium (Botanic Gardens), the Departments of Agriculture or Primary Industry, or the Safety Centre in your state.

annual — lasts one year
biennial — lasts two years
deciduous — shed leaves every year
evergreen — has leaves all throughout the year
herbaceous — fleshy plants
perennial — a long time

Common name	Botanical name	Identifying features
Angel's Trumpet Datura	*Brugmansia* x *candida* (previously known as *Datura* x *candida*, *D. arborea* or *D. suaveolens*)	Large evergreen shrub with large, soft, hairy broad leaves; large white, cream or apricot trumpet flowers to 25 cm. Commonly grown in gardens.
Arum Lily Calla Lily Death Lily Garden Calla	*Zantedeschia* *aethiopica*	Fleshy perennial with large, soft arrow-shaped leaves; fleshy, golden, finger-like rod of flower parts to 10 cm, almost wrapped in a large white fleshy leaf.Often found near creeks or in boggy soil.
Castor Bean Castor Oil Plant	*Ricinis communis*	Tall annual to 3 m; large, broad, leaves up to 75 cm, in the shape of a person's hand (young, leaves are pink or reddish, old leaves are green); seeds in spiky seed heads. Often grows in waste areas.
Daffodil Jonquil Narcissus Paperwhite	*Narcissus* species	Bulbs with long and thin leaves; single or small groups of yellow, cream or white trumpet-shaped flowers on stem. Bulbs are often stored in the refrigerator.
Deadly Nightshade	*Atropa belladonna*	Herbaceous perennial with small, purplish, bell-shaped flowers to 5 cm, arranged singly along the stem; glossy, dark purple-black berries contain many seeds. Found in waste places and along roadsides.
Dieffenbachia Dumb Plant Dumbcane	*Dieffenbachia* species	Soft-stemmed perennial with large oval leaves to 30 cm; often spotted or blotched with white, cream or yellow. Common indoor plant in homes and public settings.
Digitalis Fairy Bells Foxglove	*Digitalis purpurea*	Biennial with tall flowering stems to 1 m; flowers are bell-shaped, often white, pink or purple with prominent black spots. A common spring cottage-garden plant, sold as seedlings from punnets.
Lantana	*Lantana camara*	Evergreen shrub to 3 m, with rough leaves and slightly prickly stems. Small, tubular, pink flowers that turn cream and yellow; green berries turn black as they mature (cultivated forms do not usually produce berries).The wild form is a weed, and invades natural bushland.

Poisonous parts	Toxicity rating	Possible symptoms
All parts, particularly leaves and flowers	Extreme	Dry mouth, hallucinations, heart rate increases; death.
All parts contain a poisonous sap	Extreme	Swelling of the lips, mouth and throat (and other mucous membranes), causing difficulty in breathing; death.
Small quantities of chewed seeds; possibly leaves	Extreme	Prompt burning sensation in the mouth and throat, headache, abdominal pain. Nausea and vomiting (may be delayed); death. Seeds can also cause an itching skin allergy.
Bulbs, stems, leaves	Moderate	Skin rashes in some cases; nausea, vomiting, diarrhoea (leading to dehydration), trembling, convulsions; death.
All parts, particularly berries	Extreme	Pupils dilate, difficulty in swallowing, heartbeat increases, trembling, coma; death. Poisonings are rare.
Leaves, stems, sap	Usually moderate	Swelling and blistering of eyes, mouth and throat. Immediate pain can be extreme, and swelling may cause difficulty in breathing. The immediate pain in the mouth usually means that the plant is spat out and death is rare.
Whole plant, particularly flowers and seeds	Usually moderate	Burning sensation in the mouth and throat; nausea, vomiting, abdominal pain, disrupted vision; slow, strong heartbeat; death is rare.
Leaves and green berries; leaves also cause skin allergies.	Extreme	Stomach pains, vomiting, diarrhoea, weakness; death.

Common name	Botanical name	Identifying features
Oleander Common Oleander	*Nerium oleander*	Evergreen shrub to 3 m; thick, long, leathery leaves to 20 cm; tubular white, apricot, pink, or crimson flowers, opening flat at the tip. Commonly found in gardens, on streets and other public settings.
Philodendron Heart-leaf Philodendron	*Philodendron* species, including *P. scandens*, *P. selloum*, *P. cordatum* and *P. oxycardium*	Evergreen climbers with aerial roots; large heart-shaped or arrow-shaped, glossy, dark-green leaves, can be red or green splashed with cream. Common indoor plant in homes and public settings.
Rhus Scarlet Rhus Sumac Wax Tree	*Rhus succedanea* (formerly known as *Toxicodendron succedaneum*)	Small deciduous tree; leaves of up to 15 leaflets change from green to scarlet; masses of light-brown, single-seeded berries on female trees during autumn after the leaves fall. Common garden plant.
Poinsettia Christmas Flower	*Euphorbia pulcherrima*	Evergreen small shrub; large leaves withr broadly-toothed edges; red upper leaves; cream and pink cultivated forms now available. Common indoor plant in homes and public settings.
White Cedar Cape Lilac Chinaberry Tree	*Melia azedarach* (formerly known as *M. azedarach* var. *australasica*)	Small deciduous tree; large leaves of many leaflets; mauve flowers, followed by one-seeded green fruit that turn yellow then a wrinkled orange, remaining on the tree after leaf fall. Frequently planted as a street tree in country towns for its extreme resistance to drought.
Wisteria Chinese Wisteria Japanese Wisteria	*Wisteria floribunda*, *W. sinensis*	Deciduous climber; leaves of many leaflets, mauve, pink or white pendulous pea flowers, followed by hairy pods. Japanese Wisteria flowers may reach 1 m; Chinese Wisteria flowers are shorter, to 25 cm, and fragrant. Very common garden plant.
Yellow Oleander Lucky Nut Tree Daffodil	*Thevetia peruviana*	Evergreen shrub to 4 m; narrow, shiny, bright green leaves; stems contain a milky sap; clear yellow to orange, tubular flowers opening to flat lobes; green and fleshy fruit, ripens to yellow, then black; brown, triangular seeds are often found on the ground below the plant. Widely used as a garden plant in tropical areas; naturalised in coastal Qld and NSW.

Poisonous parts	Toxicity rating	Possible symptoms
All parts; as well as vase water, honey made from flowers, and smoke from burning	Extreme	Pain in the mouth and throat; dizziness, vomiting, diarrhoea, slowed heartbeat, irregular heartbeat; death. Death is uncommon, as the sap is very bitter tasting and the plant is spat out. Skin allergies are common.
Leaves, stems and roots	Moderate	Pain, swelling of lips, mouth and throat (and other mucous membranes). Immediate discomfort usually means that the plant is spat out, and death is rare.
All parts, especially leaves	Moderate	Contact with the plant may cause an allergic reaction. Pain, itchiness, swelling, blistering, possibly requiring hospitalisation.
All parts contain irritant sap	Mild	Allergic skin reactions can appear after contact with the sap; stinging and blistering of the lips; harmless if swallowed.
Fruit and seed	Moderate	Severe abdominal pain, nausea, severe thirst, cold sweats, bloody diarrhoea, vomiting; sleepiness, convulsions; death. The fruit has a bad odour and taste, so death is rare.
Pods and seeds	Mild	Abdominal pain, vomiting, dehydration. Full recovery usually occurs within 24 hours.
All parts, especially flowers, seeds, leaves	Extreme	Sharp, bitter burning sensation in the mouth; lips may become numb. Nausea, severe vomiting and diarrhoea may occur after some hours, slowed heartbeat, heart failure; death. One chewed and swallowed seed is enough to kill a child.

Teeth injuries

Facts

First teeth or primary teeth, usually appear at about 6 to 9 months of age, although some babies have them from birth. By about 2 or 3 years a child will have 20 teeth. Gradually these primary teeth fall out, and are replaced by permanent or secondary teeth. This may start to happen when a child is about 6 years old. By 12 years of age children will have most of their permanent teeth.

Injuries to primary teeth most commonly result from falls, car accidents and play equipment. They include: broken teeth, teeth knocked out, teeth partially dislodged, or teeth pushed up into the gum. Older children, particularly boys over 8 years, are more likely to have a permanent tooth knocked out, partially dislodged or broken during sport, bicycling, skateboarding, or when playing rough games with others. Sometimes injuries to the teeth may be associated with cuts and/or abrasions to the face, lips, gums or other part of the mouth.

Regular dental checkups are recommended from 12 months of age so that parents can be given preventive dental health information. Earlier dental checkups may be necessary for medical reasons.

Prevention

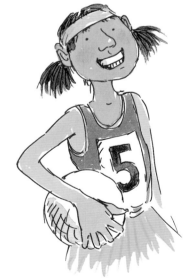

- A sports mouthguard, which can be fitted by a dentist, reduces the risk of injury to the front teeth, jaws, lips and tongue. It should be worn by a child when practising and playing contact or ball sports such as football, soccer, netball, basketball or hockey. Similarly, children should wear protective headgear when practising or playing cricket.
- When travelling by car, make sure your child is properly restrained at all times. See **Safety in the car** (pp. 12–14) and **Traffic accidents** (p. 113).

Wear a professionally fitted mouthguard.

First aid

Tooth knocked out

If a second or permanent tooth is knocked out, it should always be replaced in the mouth if possible. Immediate replacement of the tooth and early dental treatment often results in the tooth surviving.

What to do

1 *If possible, find the tooth.*

2 *Decide whether the tooth is a primary or secondary tooth:*
- *If the child is 6 years or less, it is likely to be a primary tooth.*
- *If the child is 7 years or more, it is likely to be a secondary tooth.*
If you are unsure whether it is a primary or a secondary tooth:
- *Place it in a container of milk.*
- *Immediately take the child and the tooth to a dentist, dental hospital, or hospital emergency department. If possible, call the dentist before you visit to advise that you are on your way there, and follow any advice that is given.*

3 *If the lost tooth is a primary tooth:*
- *Do not replace it in the mouth.*
- *Take the child immediately to a dentist, dental hospital or hospital emergency department. If possible, call the dentist before you visit to advise that you are on your way there, and follow any advice that is given.*

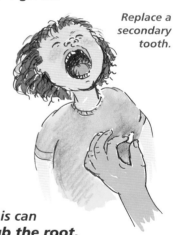
Replace a secondary tooth.

If the lost tooth is a secondary tooth:
- *Gently rinse it in milk, or if readily available a commercially produced saline solution. Never use water, as this can damage the tooth's root. **Do not scrub the root.***
- *Immediately put the rinsed tooth back into the socket, being careful to place it the right way around.*
- *If you cannot easily replace the tooth because of damage to the mouth, or because the child won't co-operate, it is important to place it in a small amount of milk in a suitable container to stop the tooth from drying out. If this is not possible, place it in a commercially produced saline solution, or wrap it in some cling wrap. As a last resort, wrap it in a handkerchief dampened with the child's saliva.*

- *Take the child and the tooth immediately to a dentist, dental hospital or hospital emergency department. If possible, call the dentist before you visit to advise that you are on your way there, and follow any advice that is given.*

Tooth partially dislodged

What to do

1 *If the tooth is partially dislodged, loose, or pushed up into the gum, do not touch it or try to move it.*

2 *Take the child immediately to a dentist, dental hospital or hospital emergency department. If possible, call the dentist before you visit to advise that you are on your way there, and follow any advice that is given.*

Broken (fractured) tooth

What to do

1 *If the tooth is fractured, try to find the missing piece or pieces.*

2 *If found, try to keep the piece or pieces moist. Place it in a small amount of milk in a suitable container to stop it drying out. If this is not possible, place it in a commercially produced saline solution, or wrap it in some cling wrap. As a last resort, wrap it in a handkerchief dampened with the child's saliva.*

3 *Take the child and the piece or pieces immediately to a dentist, dental hospital or hospital emergency department. If possible, call the dentist before you visit to advise that you are on your way there, and follow any advice that is given.*

Bleeding inside the mouth

Minor bleeding inside the mouth following a dental injury will usually stop without assistance within a few minutes. If the bleeding continues for longer than this, or if there is a lot of bleeding, follow these steps.

What to do

1 *Control the bleeding by applying gentle pressure with a clean cloth, such as a piece of gauze or a face washer.*

2 *Take the child immediately to a dentist, dental hospital or hospital emergency department. If possible, call the dentist before you visit to advise that you are on your way there, and follow any advice that is given.*

Traffic accidents

Facts

There has been a steady decrease in road deaths throughout Australia in the last twenty years. This is the result of the introduction of laws making it compulsory to wear seat belts, use child restraints and wear bicycle helmets, as well as random alcohol breath testing and speed cameras in some Australian states. Car designs and roadways have become safer, and there are more public awareness campaigns promoting safe behaviour.

Despite this improvement, hundreds of children die or are badly injured each year. Children under 5 years of age are most at risk as passengers, children between 5 and 9 years as pedestrians, and older children as cyclists.

Some children will survive a car crash, but die from a blocked airway or from bleeding. Your calm and quick action at the scene of an accident may save a child's or another person's life.

Prevention

Passengers: safety in the car

Children must be placed in a car restraint suitable for their size, weight and age, and which is properly installed; see **Safety in the car** (pp. 12–15). Even in low-speed crashes a child can be injured if not properly restrained.

- The back seat is the safest for children.
- A toddler will sometimes get restless, and try to undo the harness. You must discourage the child from doing so. Pull over to the kerb, and readjust the harness. Remember to reward and praise your child every time the child keeps it on.
- Children with a medical condition or a physical disability may need a specially designed seat. Talk to an occupational therapist, physiotherapist or safety consultant at your nearest Children's Hospital about the best option.
- On long trips plan plenty of stops, and activities such as 'I spy' for children to do in the car.
- Make sure there are no loose objects on the parcel shelf, seat or floor of the car that could fly about in a crash and cause injuries.

Pedestrians: safety when crossing roads

Children under 9 years do not have the skills or abilities to cross roads safely on their own. They are easily distracted, often misjudge the distance and speed of cars, and do not make the best use of their vision and hearing.

- Always hold the hand of your child when near or crossing the road.
- A child learns by example. Use traffic lights or a pedestrian crossing when they are available.
- Teach your child to 'Stop, Look, Listen, and Think' before and while crossing roads. Choose a safe place to cross a road, where you and your child have a clear view of the road, and can be clearly seen by drivers.
- If your child takes a ball to school, make sure it stays in the school bag until the child gets to school.

Bicycle passengers: safety on the back of a bicycle

Child bicycle seats on the back of bikes are becoming increasingly popular. If you ride a bike and plan to carry your child with you, follow these guidelines:

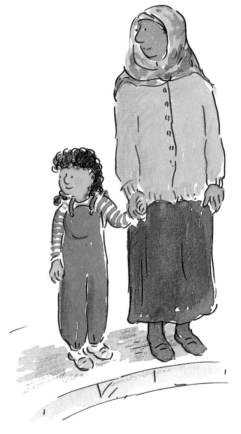

Hold your child's hand when crossing the road.

- Your child should preferably be over 12 months of age, and weigh no more than 22 kg.
- Choose a child's bike seat with head and neck support, feet straps, a full-body safety harness, moulded leg frame and spoke shields.
- Avoid roads, and use bike paths.
- You and your child should wear properly fitted Standards Australia approved bicycle helmets.

Cyclists: safety on the road

- A young child riding a tricycle in the backyard should also wear a helmet.
- Involve your child in choosing a bicycle helmet, and the child is more likely to want to wear it. There are many lightweight, well-ventilated, bright and colourful ones appealing to and suitable for children.
- Children under 9 years should not ride a bicycle unsupervised on the road or at night.

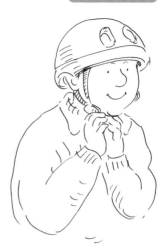

First aid

What to do

While very few of us can imagine being the first one at the scene of an accident, it is always a possibility. Learn and revise these techniques regularly, so that you are prepared to help injured children or adults.

Keep a first aid kit in your car in the event of an emergency.

These are the steps you need to follow:

1   *Make the area safe.*

2   *Turn off the ignition of the crashed vehicle.*

3   *Get help from others to warn approaching cars, and to call an ambulance and the police.*

4   *Make sure people do not smoke, as there could be petrol on the road.*

5   *If the vehicle has crashed into a power pole and wires are down, do not go near it or try to rescue someone from the vehicle, as you risk your own life.*

6   *Help any injured people; and look around quickly for anyone else who may be injured. If possible, ask the driver if there are any other passengers such as babies or small children who may have been thrown out or still inside the vehicle. Make sure someone has called an ambulance.*

7   *Remove all people from the vehicle. If weather conditions are harsh or an injured person has painful leg injuries, the person may need to be left in the vehicle.*

8 *If the person is conscious, assist the person from the vehicle. Get others to help if possible. Support any injured limbs, and try not to twist the person's neck or back. Place the person in a comfortable position or on the side.*

If a conscious person is trapped in the vehicle, try to get the person to lie on the side. Reassure and stay with the person until an ambulance arrives.

9 *If the person is unconscious, remove the person from the vehicle carefully. Get others to help if possible. Try not to twist the neck or back when moving an injured person. Follow the* **Life-threatening emergencies chart** *(front flap) until an ambulance arrives.*

If an unconscious person is trapped in the vehicle, clear the airway of any blood and vomit, and then tilt the head and lift the jaw. If necessary you can give mouth-to-mouth resuscitation to someone sitting in a vehicle; however, the person must be removed from the vehicle before you perform CPR.

10 *Stop bleeding by applying firm pressure to any wounds, using a clean cloth, towel or other bulky material. Avoid contact with blood, if possible, by using rubber gloves, or a plastic bag, or other similar material. If you come in contact with blood, wash it off immediately with soap and water.*

11 *Help an injured person support a fractured limb in a comfortable position to reduce pain until the ambulance arrives.*

Illnesses

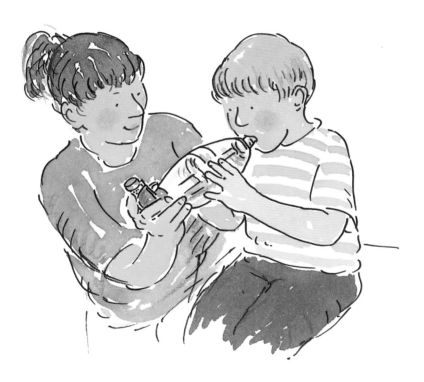

Asthma

Facts

Asthma is a common condition affecting one in four Australian children. A child with asthma has more sensitive airways than normal. When these airways are exposed to a 'trigger' they can overreact and narrow, causing an asthma attack.

Children may have only occasional asthma attacks, lasting 2–10 days, and they may be brought on by a cold. Other children have frequent attacks every 4–6 weeks, while some have an attack or wheeze almost every day. These attacks might be mild, moderate or severe.

It isn't clear why some children develop asthma. It may be inherited, especially if someone else in the family has asthma, hayfever or allergies. Children who are exposed to cigarette smoke at an early age seem to be at greater risk of developing asthma.

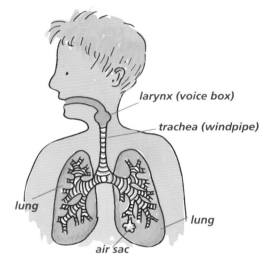

larynx (voice box)

trachea (windpipe)

lung

lung

air sac

extra mucus

normal airway

airway narrowed during an asthma attack

Prevention

You can't really prevent asthma, but by understanding the condition and how to treat it correctly you may reduce the number and severity of attacks.

Knowing and avoiding triggers

A number of different triggers can bring on an asthma attack. These include colds and viruses, exercise, emotional upset, pollens, dust, tobacco smoke, animal hair, and a change in temperature, particularly moving into cold air.

Triggers can differ with each child, and there may be more than one trigger. Knowing and avoiding triggers can reduce the chances of a sudden attack.

Proper use of medications

Two main groups of medications are used to treat asthma. These are known as preventers and relievers.

Preventers need to be taken regularly in order to decrease the number and severity of attacks. They work by reducing the swelling in the airways, and include Becloforte, Becotide, Pulmicort, Intal and Intal Forte. They are available in brown, beige, yellow or white containers, and as aerosol inhalers (puffers) and dry powder inhalers. Preventers don't help during a sudden asthma attack.

Relievers work quickly to make breathing easier. They include Ventolin, Respolin, Bricanyl and Asmol. They are available as aerosol inhalers (puffers), dry powder inhalers, or in a solution form for use with a nebuliser pump. The puffers are commonly in blue, grey or green containers.

Children under 8 years usually need to use a puffer or inhaler with a spacer device, or a power-driven nebuliser. A spacer device is placed between the puffer and the child's mouth to hold the asthma medication; it ensures that the child receives all of the medication. A nebuliser breaks down the asthma medication into a fine mist, which the child breaths in through a mask. Nebulisers are particularly useful for children with frequent or severe asthma.

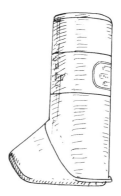
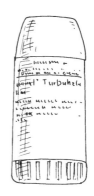
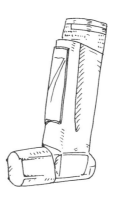

Asthma medications.

Exercise and asthma

A child with asthma should be encouraged to exercise and participate in sport. Sports such as prolonged running may dry out the airways and cause an asthma attack. Sometimes if a child takes Intal, or a reliever medication such as Ventolin, 5–10 minutes before exercise this may prevent an attack. Discuss this with your doctor.

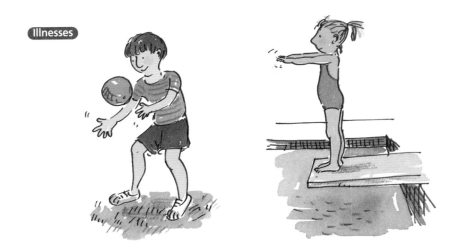

Swimming is one of the best types of exercise for children with asthma. While swimming, the child breathes in air that is moist and less likely to cause an attack, particularly if the pool is heated.

Understanding asthma treatment

A child with asthma should have regular check-ups, and develop a personal asthma action plan with the family doctor. This action plan will help the child and parent to better understand and manage the asthma. It also indicates if the asthma is getting worse, how to treat an attack quickly, and when to see a doctor.

It is important to understand that even a child with well-controlled asthma can have a serious life-threatening attack without warning. No asthma attack should be left untreated, even mild ones. If not treated, an attack may quickly become life-threatening.

First aid

What to look for
➤ wheezing (in severe attacks it might not be heard)
➤ coughing (may be the only sign of asthma, particularly at night)
➤ breathing more quickly than normal, and using greater effort
➤ tightness in the chest
➤ difficulty speaking
➤ the child may be pale, and have a fast pulse.

What to do
Follow the child's personal asthma action plan. If medication is normally given via a nebuliser pump, follow the usual procedure. **Do not use dry powder inhalers and syrups in an emergency**.

If an action plan is not available, follow these steps:

1 *Reassure the child. Take the child to a warm, quiet area to rest.*

2 *Help the child take 4 puffs of reliever medication (aerosol inhaler). This is best given through a spacer device. Shake the puffer, and give 2 puffs into the spacer at a time. Ask the child to breathe in and out of the spacer 4–5 times.*

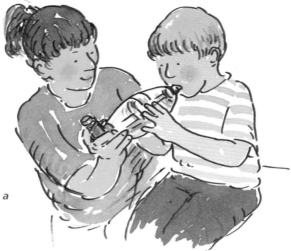

Reliever medication given through a spacer device.

3 *Wait 4 minutes. If there is no improvement, give the child another 4 puffs of reliever medication, as above.*

4 *If there is still no improvement, call an ambulance immediately.*

5 *Continue giving 4 puffs of reliever medication every 4 minutes while waiting for the ambulance.*
    Always call an ambulance immediately if the child is unable to take the medication, if the condition suddenly gets worse, or if you are concerned at any time.

6 *If the child becomes unconscious, follow the **Life-threatening emergencies chart** (front flap), and call an ambulance. If the child stops breathing, use **mouth-to-mouth resuscitation** (see pp. 30-1). Because air can be trapped in the lungs, resuscitation breaths should be given more slowly (every 6 seconds).*

For further information about asthma, contact the Asthma Foundation in your state or territory.

Croup

Facts

Viral infections can cause croup. The child's windpipe becomes inflamed and narrows. This results in breathing difficulties and a barking type of cough. Croup is a common condition usually affecting children under 3 years of age, but may occur in older children.

Unlike epiglottitis, croup develops slowly; see **Epiglottitis** (p. 127). Normally croup won't be severe enough to require medical treatment, and the child gets better in a few days. Antibiotics don't help. Only occasionally does croup become so severe that the child requires emergency treatment.

Prevention

Apart from taking a sensible approach to avoiding the 'winter chills or ills', little can be done to prevent croup.

First aid

What to look for
➤ a cold or a runny nose
➤ possibly a mild fever
➤ a sore and hoarse throat
➤ a harsh, high-pitched sound when breathing in (worse at night)

➤ a barking or hacking cough (worse at night)
➤ restlessness and irritability.

What to do
A child waking up with croup may be quite distressed.

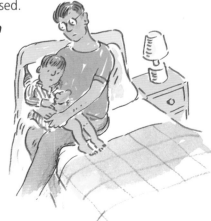

1 *In most cases the child will settle with gentle reassurance and a cuddle. Sometimes caring for the child in a warm, humid environment, such as a steam-filled bathroom, may help.*

2 *If the child won't settle or is having any difficulty breathing, call an ambulance.*

3 *If the child becomes unconscious, follow the Life-threatening emergencies chart (front flap), and call an ambulance.*

122

Dehydration

Facts

A child can become dehydrated quickly if too much body fluid is lost and not replaced. This may be caused by gastroenteritis, a viral infection that causes vomiting and diarrhoea, an illness where a child won't or can't drink, or exposure to very hot conditions.

Prevention

Infections such as gastroenteritis can spread easily and quickly. If a member of the family has diarrhoea or has been vomiting, make sure that everyone washes their hands before eating or drinking, or after going to the toilet. If the baby has the infection, wash your hands after changing a nappy.

Babies and young children do not cope well in hot weather, and can dehydrate quickly. See **Over-exposure to heat** (p. 138) and **Heat exhaustion and heat stroke** (p. 139).

First aid

What to look for
➤ passes urine less often
➤ eyes look dark or sunken
➤ mouth and tongue dry
➤ paleness
➤ tired
➤ loss of weight.

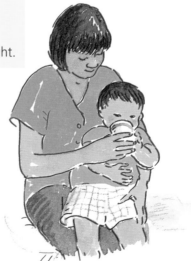

What to do

1 *Give a sick baby or child extra water.*

2 *Consult a doctor if vomiting or diarrhoea continues, or the child shows any signs of dehydration.*

See also **Heat exhaustion and heat stroke** (p. 139).

Give extra water.

123

Diabetic emergencies

Facts

A child needs glucose (a type of sugar) for energy and growth. Insulin is produced in the pancreas and travels in the bloodstream; it helps the body to make use of glucose.

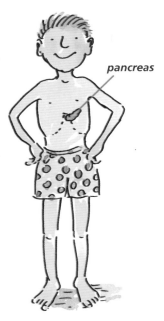

pancreas

A child with diabetes does not make enough insulin. Without it, glucose builds up in the blood. Insulin injections will be needed daily throughout life to balance the sugar levels in the blood. This condition is known as Type I diabetes, juvenile-onset or insulin-dependent diabetes.

A diabetic emergency can happen when the blood-sugar levels become too high or too low. Both these conditions can be life-threatening. Low blood-sugar can develop within minutes, whereas high blood-sugar develops slowly, usually over several days. With such early warning, high blood-sugar can be easily and quickly treated, and is unlikely to become serious. An emergency is more likely to occur because of low blood-sugar.

Prevention

It is not clear why some children develop diabetes. To keep in good health a child with diabetes will need to find the right balance between diet (a source of glucose), exercise (which uses up glucose) and insulin. Regular medical check-ups and changes to insulin levels and diet will be needed as the child grows.

Low blood-sugar (hypoglycaemia or 'hypo')

Low blood-sugar can result if a child has had too big a dose of insulin, or not enough food for the insulin to work on. It can sometimes happen when a child has been ill, under stress or during exercise. With too much insulin, sugar levels fall quickly.

124

- Meals should not be missed or delayed.
- Extra sugar should be carried at all times.
- Extra food and sugar will be needed before exercise.

High blood-sugar (hyperglycaemia)

This can result from a child not having an insulin injection, eating too much or the wrong type of food, or because of illness and stress.

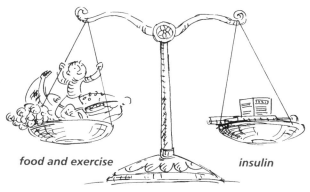

food and exercise   *insulin*

- A child with diabetes must learn to keep to a special diet. Sometimes a child may find it hard to resist an offer of sweets (other than diabetic sweets), chocolates, cakes or biscuits. Explain to other parents, carers and teachers the importance of discouraging children and adults from offering such foods to your child.

First aid

Low blood-sugar

What to look for
➤ the child complains of hunger
➤ faintness and dizziness
➤ weak and tired
➤ confusion and drowsiness
➤ sudden change in behaviour
➤ irritability, temper tantrums or aggressiveness

➤ headache
➤ pale and sweating
➤ convulsions
➤ unconsciousness.

What to do

1 *If the child is unconscious, follow the **Life-threatening emergencies chart** (front flap), and call an ambulance. Do not give anything to eat or drink, as this can enter the airway.*

If the child is conscious, give some food or a drink with sugar in it, such as a few pieces of barley sugar or chocolate, 5–7 jelly beans, 2–3 teaspoons of honey, a glass of lemonade, or water sweetened with 2 teaspoons of sugar.

125

2 *The child should feel better in 5–10 minutes as the blood-sugar level rises. Once the child improves, give some food, such as a sandwich, biscuits or fruit.*

3 *If the child's condition doesn't improve, call an ambulance. Do not give an insulin injection, as this will make the condition worse.*

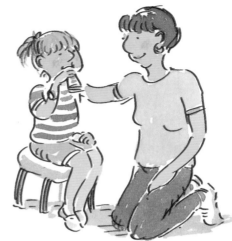

Treating low blood-sugar.

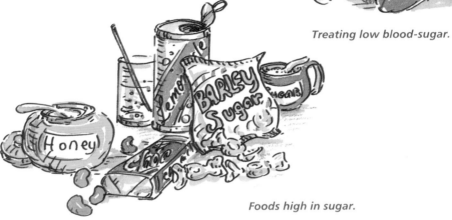

Foods high in sugar.

High blood-sugar

What to look for
➤ very thirsty
➤ tired
➤ needs to urinate often
➤ rapid pulse
➤ sweet sickly smell on breath
➤ flushed face, dry mouth and skin
➤ stomach ache
➤ vomiting and nausea
➤ unconsciousness (rare).

What to do

1 *If you think a child has high blood-sugar, take the child to a doctor urgently.*

2 *If the child becomes unconscious, follow the **Life-threatening emergencies chart** (front flap), and call an ambulance.*

126

Epiglottitis

Facts

The epiglottis is like a 'trapdoor' at the back of the throat that stops food from entering the child's windpipe when swallowing. Occasionally it can become infected, resulting in swelling and narrowing of the airway. This is known as epiglottitis, and is caused by the germ *Haemophilus influenzae* type b (Hib) (see p. 132).

Epiglottitis develops suddenly and rapidly, sometimes within a few hours. It usually affects children between 2 and 5 years, and can be life-threatening.

Prevention

All children under 5 years can and should be immunised against *Haemophilus influenzae*. Vaccination can be started at 2 months of age. For information, contact your maternal and child health nurse, local council, community health centre or a doctor. See **Infectious diseases** (p. 130).

First aid

What to look for
➤ fever
➤ lethargy
➤ the child is pale and looks unwell
➤ the child is distressed and restless
➤ difficulty breathing, making soft snoring sounds
➤ excessive salivation and drooling.

What to do

1 *If you suspect epiglottitis, sit the child up, and avoid excessive handling. Never lie the child flat or attempt to look into the mouth.*

2 *Call an ambulance.*

3 *If the child becomes unconscious, follow the **Life-threatening emergencies chart** (front flap), and call an ambulance.*

Infectious diseases

Facts

Many childhood infectious diseases spread quickly. The infections differ in severity; for example, whooping cough may result in your child being very sick, whereas school sores will cause minor discomfort.

Some infectious diseases can be prevented by immunisation — that is, by building up your child's body's defence against these diseases through vaccination. Some vaccinations have to be given several times to achieve maximum protection.

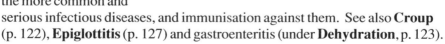

The spread of diseases can also be reduced by limiting your child's contact with another child who may have an infection; by making sure that proper hygiene practices are always maintained, such as all members of the family washing hands before eating or handling food, after going to the toilet, or wiping a runny nose.

This chapter gives information on some of the more common and serious infectious diseases, and immunisation against them. See also **Croup** (p. 122), **Epiglottitis** (p. 127) and gastroenteritis (under **Dehydration**, p. 123).

Prevention

Immunisation
Take your baby or child to a local government clinic, a community health centre, maternal and child health nurse or doctor to receive the vaccinations.

The vaccine is given by an injection or, in the case of polio, liquid drops by mouth. When vaccinated, the child's body makes antibodies that fight the disease; this is called an immune response. If the child comes into contact with the disease later, the child is better protected, and less likely to catch the disease.

Children should be immunised against the following infectious diseases, starting when a child is 2 months of age:

diphtheria	polio (poliomyelitis)
Haemophilus influenzae type b	rubella (German measles)
measles	tetanus
mumps	whooping cough (pertussis)

See the immunisation table on p. 130. Vaccinations may be delayed on medical advice on rare occasions. It is best to check with your doctor or maternal and child health nurse if you are unsure about your baby's health on an immunisation day.

When a child is immunised, there may be some minor side-effects such as fever; irritability; or redness, swelling, soreness, itching or burning at the site of the injection. Ask what to expect with each vaccination and seek medical advice if you are concerned. These side-effects are minor compared to having the disease, and will last for only a short time. Serious side-effects are rare. Before immunisation, give your child a dose of paracetamol, according to the instructions on the bottle, and every 4–6 hours (up to 24 hours) after immunisation to reduce these effects.

Children must be vaccinated at specific ages to ensure that they are protected from diseases as much as possible. Many child-care centres and schools require an immunisation certificate or record of a child's immunisation history before the child can be enrolled. If there is an outbreak of a disease, children who have not been immunised against it may be required to be kept at home.

Any child under 5 years who may have missed out on vaccinations at the specified ages can still be immunised; see your maternal and child health nurse or doctor for advice.

Children can also be immunised against hepatitis B. Discuss this with your maternal and child health nurse or immunisation provider. It is given in a schedule of 0, 1 and 6 months for babies and children up to 10 years where a mother is a hepatitis B carrier, or if they belong to ethnic groups in which the hepatitis carrier rate exceeds 2 per cent.

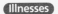

Immunisation schedule

(based on the National Health and Medical Research Council (NHMRC) Childhood Immunisation Schedule as recommended by the Department of Human Services, Victoria)

Age	Immunisation
2 months	Triple antigen, for diphtheria, tetanus and whooping cough Sabin (oral), for polio HibTITER, for *Haemophilus influenzae* type b
4 months	Triple antigen, for diphtheria, tetanus and whooping cough Sabin (oral), for polio HibTITER, for *Haemophilus influenzae* type b
6 months	Triple antigen, for diphtheria, tetanus and whooping cough Sabin (oral), for polio HibTITER, for *Haemophilus influenzae* type b
12 months	MMR, for measles, mumps and rubella
18 months	Triple antigen, for diphtheria, tetanus and whooping cough HibTITER, for *Haemophilus influenzae* type b
5 years or before starting school	Triple antigen, for diphtheria, tetanus and whooping cough Sabin (oral), for polio
10–16 years	MMR, for measles, mumps and rubella
15 years or before leaving school	ADT, for diphtheria and tetanus (adult vaccine) Sabin (oral) for polio

Australian Aborigines and Torres Strait Islanders should receive PedvaxHIB at 2, 4 and 12 months instead of HibTITER for *Haemophilus influenzae* type b.

First aid

Chickenpox

Chickenpox is caused by a virus that results in spots, then blisters, over the child's body. It spreads easily and quickly by coughing, or by contact with the spots or blisters. A child with chickenpox is infectious from a few days before the spots appear until all the blisters have turned into scabs. The fluid under the blisters and scabs is infectious.

What to look for

Before spots appear:
➤ fever
➤ runny nose
➤ coughing and sneezing
➤ tiredness

followed by:
➤ small red spots that are itchy and turn into blisters, then scabs, after a few days.

What to do

1. *Soothe the child's itchy skin by dabbing calamine lotion on the blisters or scabs, and firmly discourage the child from scratching as this can make the condition worse and the blisters and scabs may become infected. Cut the child's fingernails; or place gloves or socks on the child's hands. A soothing lotion may be added to the bath water; ask your chemist for advice.*

2. *To reduce discomfort, give the child paracetamol according to the instructions on the bottle.*

3. *If the child is distressed by the itchiness, take the child to a doctor.*

4. *To prevent the spread of the infection, teach your child to cover the mouth with a tissue when coughing; to wash hands before eating or handling food, or after blowing the nose; and keep your child away from others, in particular adults who have not had chickenpox, and pregnant women. Don't allow the child to share eating utensils.*

Common cold

During winter, preschoolers, in particular, often get colds, which can last for several days or a week or more. Colds are caused by many different viruses.

What to look for

➤ coughing and sneezing
➤ a runny nose
➤ sore throat
➤ headache

➤ fever
➤ irritability
➤ loss of appetite.

What to do

1 *Try to make the child as comfortable as possible. Bed rest is not necessary unless the child is particularly unwell. Encourage your child to play quietly inside if it is cold outdoors, but don't overheat the child.*

2 *Give your child plenty to drink. To reduce discomfort, give a dose of paracetamol according to the instructions on the bottle.*

3 *If your child's condition does not improve in a couple of days, or if the child has difficulty breathing, refuses to eat or drink, has sore ears, starts to vomit, or if you are concerned, take the child to a doctor.*

4 *To prevent the spread of infection, teach your child to cover the mouth with a tissue when coughing; to wash hands before eating or handling food, or after blowing the nose. Don't allow the child to share eating utensils.*

Haemophilus influenzae type b (Hib)

Hib is a bacterium living in the nose and throat, and can result in serious life-threatening infections such as meningitis, pneumonia, joint infection, infection under the skin, or epiglottitis (see **Epiglottitis**, p.127). Children under 5 years are most at risk of serious infections, and should be immunised against Hib.

What to look for

➤ high fever
➤ vomiting
➤ headache
➤ irritability

➤ difficulty swallowing or breathing
➤ convulsions or fits
➤ stiffness in the neck.

What to do

1 *If the child shows these signs, or if you are at all concerned, take the child to a doctor immediately.*

2 *If the child loses consciousness or is having trouble breathing, follow the **Life-threatening emergencies chart** (front flap), and call an ambulance.*

Hand, foot and mouth disease

This infection, common among preschoolers, is caused by a virus. The infection is usually not serious, and is spread through contact with the moist blisters on the child's body, and with faeces. Hand, foot and mouth disease is not the same as foot/hoof and mouth disease occurring in some animals.

What to look for
➤ blisters in the mouth, on the hands and feet, lasting 7–10 days
➤ red spots on the buttocks
➤ fever
➤ listlessness
➤ loss of appetite.

What to do

1 *Give your child plenty of fluids. If blisters in the mouth make it difficult for the child to eat, give the child soft or liquid foods. Avoid acidic foods such as oranges or tomatoes, which will cause pain.*

2 *To reduce discomfort, give the child paracetamol according to the instructions on the bottle.*

3 *If your child refuses to eat or drink, or if you are concerned, take the child to a doctor.*

Measles

Measles is a viral infection, spread easily through sneezing and coughing. Measles can sometimes lead to other serious secondary infections affecting the ear, lungs or brain. Children should be immunised against measles.

What to look for
➤ runny nose
➤ dry cough
➤ tiredness
➤ sore and red eyes
➤ high fever

➤ small white spots on the inside of the cheek in the mouth
➤ a red blotchy rash starting behind the ears and along the hairline, and which spreads all over the body.

What to do

1 *If you think your child may have measles, take the child to a doctor.*

2 *To reduce any discomfort, give the child paracetamol according to the instructions on the bottle.*

3 *To prevent the spread of infection, keep your child away from others for at least a week after the rash has appeared. Teach your child to cover the mouth with a tissue when coughing; to wash hands before eating or handling food, or after blowing the nose. Don't allow the child to share eating utensils.*

Mumps

Mumps is caused by a virus, and is spread by coughing and sneezing. Sometimes mumps can lead to other conditions that can affect the brain and spinal cord. Children should be immunised against mumps.

What to look for
➤ fever
➤ headache
➤ pain when chewing or swallowing, due to swollen glands
➤ in boys on rare occasions, tenderness in the testicles.

What to do

1 *If you think your child may have the mumps, take the child to a doctor.*

2 *To reduce discomfort, give your child paracetamol according to the instructions on the bottle.*

3 *If your child has difficulty swallowing, give the child soft or liquid foods.*

4 *To prevent the spread of infection, keep your child away from others for at least 9 days from the start of the swelling of the glands. Teach your child to cover the mouth with a tissue when coughing; to wash hands before eating or handling food, or after blowing the nose. Don't allow the child to share eating utensils.*

Rubella (German measles)

Rubella is a virus, and is most common in children under 13 years. Sometimes the condition is so mild that it may go unnoticed. All children should be immunised against rubella. Children born to mothers who have had rubella during pregnancy may have serious birth defects.

What to look for

➤ fever
➤ sore throat
➤ pain in joints

➤ swollen glands in the neck
➤ pink rash that starts on the face and spreads to the body.

What to do

1 *If you think your child may have rubella and is unwell, take the child to a doctor.*

2 *To reduce discomfort give your child paracetamol according to the instructions on the bottle.*

3 *To prevent the spread of infection, keep your child away from others, particularly non-immunised pregnant women, for at least a week after the rash has appeared.*

School sores (impetigo)

School sores are caused by a bacterium. The sores often appear on the face, hands and legs, and can spread quickly to other parts of the body and to other children or adults.

What to look for

➤ red blisters on the skin that turn into yellow-green scabs.

What to do

1 *Take your child to a doctor, as antibiotics may be required.*

2 *To prevent the spread of the infection:*
   • *Discourage your child from scratching, picking or touching the sores.*
   • *Keep the infected skin clean by washing with soap and water.*
   • *Cover the exposed sores with clothes or a gauze dressing (not adhesive).*
   • *Wash your child's hands, and your own, after touching sores.*
   • *Have a separate towel for your child to use.*
   • *Wash the child's towel, bed linen and clothing in hot water, separately from other washing.*
   • *Keep your child at home until treatment has started, and keep the sores covered.*

Whooping cough (pertussis)

Whooping cough is caused by a bacteria, and is spread through sneezing and coughing. It can be serious in babies and young children, and sometimes results in complications that affect the brain and lungs. All children should be immunised against whooping cough.

What to look for

➤ runny nose
➤ fever
➤ coughing, followed by vomiting
➤ breathing difficulties
➤ gasping for breath, and a high-pitched sound ('whoop') when breathing in.

What to do

1 *Calm and reassure the child. Following a coughing fit, sit the child up in case of vomiting.*

2 *The child should be seen by a doctor immediately.*

Caring for your sick child at home

Despite your efforts children still get sick. When you have to care for a child at home during a minor illness, it can be distressing and even frustrating for both parent and child, as it upsets normal routines.

The best you can do is to follow any medical advice, and try to make the child as comfortable as possible. Expect that your child will want and need extra attention. Offer plenty of reassurance, as this will soothe any unnecessary fears, help your child to be positive, and speed up the recovery process. In a few days your child will be feeling better, and so will you.

When a child is sick with a cold or other minor infection, it will not always be necessary for the child to stay in bed. Encourage your child to play quietly, watch TV, listen to the radio, draw, read or write stories. This will help to pass the time, and still allow your child to get the necessary rest. As the child's condition improves, and if the weather is reasonable, then a short walk in some fresh air is a good idea.

If your child has a reduced appetite while sick, don't be overly concerned unless the child refuses to eat or drink altogether. In this case, you should take the child to a doctor. Don't force the child to eat large amounts, and prepare a variety of simple meals and favourite foods. Make sure your child has plenty to drink, as babies and young children can dehydrate (lose water) quickly (see **Dehydration**, p. 127).

If at any time you are unsure or worried about your child's health, do not hesitate to call or take the child to a doctor, even at night!

Over-exposure to hot & cold temperatures

Facts

A child has a normal body temperature of 37°C. This temperature can vary slightly (from 36.5–37.5°C) but if it becomes very high or very low a child can become seriously ill. Children are particularly at risk of heat and cold illness because of their body size and inability to control body temperature.

A child's temperature can fall dangerously low when in cold, wet and windy conditions for a long time without any protective clothing, or after being a long time in cold water. It can become dangerously high in hot conditions, such as being left in a closed car or playing sport on a hot day. There are two types of heat illness: heat exhaustion and heat stroke. Heat stroke is more serious, and can cause brain damage and death if untreated.

Prevention

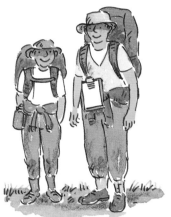

Over-exposure to cold
A little knowledge and pre-planning will ensure that children can safely enjoy such activities as bushwalking, snow-skiing and water sports.

- When camping or hiking in cold conditions, children should wear thermal underwear. Take extra warm and waterproof clothing, even on day walks, as the weather can sometimes change without warning.
- Remember to pack a hat or beanie, gloves and warm woolly socks. Heat is lost quickly from the head, hands and feet.
- Encourage children to eat and drink normally, and to take extra snacks. They should rest often to avoid getting too tired.
- Always tell someone where you plan to go and when you expect to be back. If the weather becomes bad, find shelter if possible. Carry a space blanket for emergency shelter.
- If water-skiing, snorkelling or boating, the child should wear appropriate gear, such as a wetsuit and life jacket. Teach children to keep still if lost in water to conserve body heat, or if lost in snow or fog to stop walking and find shelter.

Over-exposure to heat

Babies and young children don't cope well in hot weather. They sweat and dehydrate (lose fluids) quickly. See **Dehydration** (p. 123).

- Keep children inside on hot days. Children should play or sleep in the coolest, best-ventilated rooms. Don't overdress them. On very hot days a nappy for a baby, or underwear or shorts for older children, is enough clothing.
- If you have to go out with a child, try to do so in the early morning or early evening. Dress a child in light-coloured, loose-fitting clothing and a hat.
- Encourage the child to drink extra water or cordial, especially when playing sport.
- Children should avoid exercising or playing sport in hot humid weather.
- Never leave children (or pets) in a closed, parked car on hot days, even for a short time. The temperature inside the car may quickly rise to almost twice the temperature outside. Opening the windows slightly makes little difference.
- Young children have been known to play hide-and-seek in the boot of a car. If the car is in the driveway or garage, make sure the car doors and boot are kept locked.

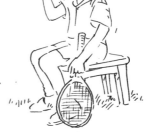

Drink extra water when playing sport.

First aid

Over-exposure to cold

What to look for
- drowsiness and confusion
- unsteadiness on feet
- shivering (may stop as the temperature gets very low)
- cool and pale skin
- slowing of pulse and breathing
- may look lifeless after a long time in the cold.

What to do

1 *If the child is unconscious, follow the **Life-threatening emergencies chart** (front flap), and call an ambulance. Keep up resuscitation until the child is in hospital or the ambulance arrives.*

2 *If the child is conscious, move the child to a dry, sheltered area. Handle gently, and keep the body straight to prevent cold blood from flowing from the arms and legs to the heart.*

3 *Remove or cut off any wet clothing, and dress the child in warm, dry clothing.*

4 *Cover the child with blankets, a space blanket or a sleeping bag; get under the covers or into the sleeping bag yourself*

to provide extra warmth for the child.
If hot water bottles are available, wrap
them in some type of cover to prevent
burns, and place them against the
child's groin, armpits and the sides of
the neck.

Warm a cold child.

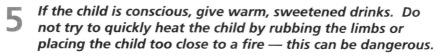

   If a shelter and warm, dry clothing
are not available, do not remove the
child's wet clothes. Wrap the child up
in whatever is available, and cover with something
waterproof to stop further heat loss.

5 If the child is conscious, give warm, sweetened drinks. Do
not try to quickly heat the child by rubbing the limbs or
placing the child too close to a fire — this can be dangerous.

6 Get the child to hospital as soon as possible, preferably by
ambulance. If transport by car is necessary, turn the car
heater on to high.

Heat exhaustion and heat stroke

What to look for
Heat exhaustion
- ➤ pale, sweaty skin
- ➤ thirst
- ➤ muscle cramps and weakness

- ➤ moderately raised body temperature
- ➤ dizziness
- ➤ confusion.

Heat stroke
- ➤ confusion
- ➤ hot, flushed dry skin
- ➤ high temperature (more than 40°C)

- ➤ rapid, pounding pulse
- ➤ unsteady on feet
- ➤ unconsciousness.

What to do
1 Lie the child down in a cool area, remove excess clothing, and
cool the child by fanning.

2 If the child is conscious, give cool water to drink.

3 If you think the child has heat stroke, wrap ice in wet cloths
and place these against the child's groin and armpits.

4 Call an ambulance. If transport by car is necessary, turn the
car airconditioner or fan on to high.

5 If the child becomes unconscious, call an ambulance and
follow the **Life-threatening emergencies chart** (front flap)
until the ambulance arrives.

Seizure, convulsion or fit

A seizure, also known as a convulsion or fit, happens when there is a sudden uncontrolled surge of electrical activity in the brain. In children this is most commonly caused by epilepsy or a high fever. Other causes can include a head injury, lack of oxygen, a brain infection, and eating poisons such as snail bait or some plants.

Epilepsy

Facts

Epilepsy may develop as a result of birth trauma, a head injury or past infections such as meningitis; in many cases the cause is unknown. The child may have recurring seizures over months or years.

There are several different types of seizures. Some seizures affect one-half of the brain (partial) or the whole of the brain (generalised). In a generalised convulsive seizure the child loses consciousness, and there is jerking and twitching of the body.

Prevention

Epilepsy cannot be prevented, but it can be controlled.

If a child has epilepsy, sometimes seizures can be triggered by:

- flashing lights
- tiredness or being 'run down'
- illness, including vomiting, diarrhoea and upper respiratory infections
- a high temperature
- over-excitement
- stress
- missed meals
- forgetting to take epilepsy medication.

Avoiding triggers, and making sure a child has a balanced approach to meals, sleep and exercise can help prevent seizures. Prescribed medication must be taken regularly.

A child with epilepsy should be encouraged to be involved in sport and recreational activities just like other children. When the child continues to have seizures:

- activities that involve climbing are not recommended
- swimming, bicycling and horse-riding require close supervision at all times.

The child should wear a special medical-alert bracelet to let others know the child has epilepsy. It is important to talk to teachers, the sports coach and other parents and carers so that they understand and know what to do if the child has a convulsion.

First aid

Generalised convulsive seizure
(a tonic-clonic seizure, previously known as grand mal)

What to look for
➤ the child becomes rigid, and falls to the ground
➤ loses consciousness
➤ twitches or jerks uncontrollably
➤ may have difficulty breathing
➤ may go blue around the lips
➤ may lose control of bladder or bowel
➤ the seizure usually lasts less than 5 minutes.

What to do

Caring for a child during a seizure.

1 Remove any objects nearby that could cause an injury, such as a table or chairs.

2 Do not try to restrain the child or put anything in the mouth.

3 Support the child's head with your hand or a soft object, such as a blanket or pillow.

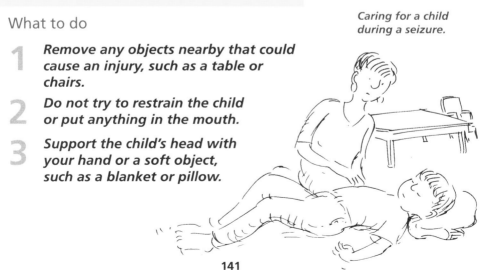

141

4 When the seizure stops, place the child on one side, and follow the **Life-threatening emergencies chart** (front flap).

5 If the child has a history of epilepsy, an ambulance usually is not needed unless the seizure lasts longer than 5 minutes, or is followed by another one. If the child has never had a seizure before, call an ambulance.

6 The child may be sleepy or confused. Reassure the child, and give a simple explanation of what has happened. Do not give any food or liquid to the child unless the child is fully awake.

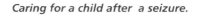

Caring for a child after a seizure.

Generalised absence seizure (previously known as petit mal) and complex partial seizure

Following these epileptic seizures, a child may wander and be confused. The child is not likely to need any first aid, but should be watched closely to avoid being injured.

What to look for

Generalised absence seizure
- ➤ brief loss of consciousness
- ➤ stares blankly
- ➤ eyelids may flutter

Partial complex seizure
- ➤ may wander
- ➤ tugs at clothes
- ➤ makes chewing movements
- ➤ hallucinates
- ➤ looks afraid and confused.

Febrile convulsion

Facts

Children can sometimes have a seizure if they develop a high fever. This is known as a febrile convulsion, and tends to occur in children under 5 years of age. It is not related to epilepsy, although the seizure is the same as a generalised (tonic-clonic) seizure. See **Generalised convulsive seizure** (pp. 141-2).

A febrile convulsion can be frightening to watch, but it is not life-threatening. There is no need for a high-speed dash to the hospital in your car.

Prevention

If you bring down a child's temperature, a febrile convulsion might be avoided; however, sometimes the convulsion is the first sign that a child has a fever.

Make sure the child is dressed in light clothing, and drinks plenty of water. If the fever is high, to reduce discomfort give paracetamol according to the instructions on the bottle. If the fever continues, consult a doctor.

First aid

What to look for
- ➤ unconsciousness
- ➤ eyes may roll back
- ➤ body may go floppy
- ➤ twitching and jerking of body.

What to do

1 **Remove any objects nearby that could cause an injury, such as a table or chairs.**

2 **Do not try to restrain the child or put anything in the mouth.**

3 **Support the child's head with your hand or a soft object, such as a blanket or pillow.**

4 **When the seizure stops, place the child on one side, and follow the Life-threatening emergencies chart (front flap).**

5 **Cool the child by removing the child's outer clothing and sponging the child down with a wet, lukewarm cloth.**

6 **Call an ambulance.**

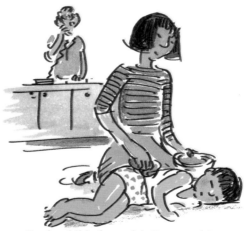

Cool a child after a febrile convulsion.

For further information about epilepsy, contact the Epilepsy Foundation in your state or territory.

Tooth decay and teething

Facts

First teeth or primary teeth, usually appear at about 6 to 9 months of age, although some babies have them from birth. By about 2 or 3 years a child will have 20 teeth. Gradually these primary teeth fall out and are replaced by permanent or secondary teeth. This may start to happen when a child is about 6 years of age. By 12 years of age children will have most of their permanent teeth.

Tooth decay occurs when the bacteria in the mouth have frequent access, or access for long periods of time, to foods containing carbohydrate. The bacteria break down the carbohydrate to produce acid, which attacks the teeth and may result in decay. Sometimes babies or toddlers develop tooth decay when:

- honey or another sweetener has been placed on the child's dummy;
- infants or toddlers drink sweet beverages such as cordial or flavoured milk from a baby bottle.

Children who are bottle fed with only milk or formula will develop tooth decay if they are left for long periods of time with the bottle in their mouth, especially at night. Even breastfeeding will cause tooth decay if the child sleeps for long periods of time while being breastfed, or if the frequency of feeds is unusually excessive.

Regular dental check-ups are recommended from 12 months of age so that parents can be given preventive dental health information. Earlier dental check-ups may be necessary for medical reasons.

Prevention

- Your baby or toddler should not be left in bed with a bottle. Bottles should not be used as a pacifier during the day.
- Don't put honey, cordial or flavoured milk in a baby's bottle or on a dummy.
- Most children can drink from a cup by 12 months of age. Once your child can do this, the use of a bottle should be discontinued.
- When your child is too young to take tablets, ask the doctor to prescribe a sugar-free syrup medicine if available.

- Clean your baby's teeth as soon as they appear by gently wiping them with a damp piece of cloth such as a face washer. Within 6 months of the arrival of the teeth you can start using a small, soft toothbrush. When a child can swish water in the mouth and spit it out, it is time to introduce toothpaste. Children up to 6 years of age should use a small amount of low-dose fluoride toothpaste (no more than the size of a pea) spread thinly along the top of the brush.
- Check if your water supply is fluoridated. If not, ask your dentist if a fluoride supplement is required for your child.
- Don't give your child sweet snacks between meals. Sticky sugar-based 'health foods' like muesli bars, health-food bars and fruit-based sticky sweets are just as likely to cause decay as other sticky sweet foods.
- Try to reduce the number of snacks your child has between meals. Give your child one large snack rather than a number of small snacks when your child is feeling hungry between meals.

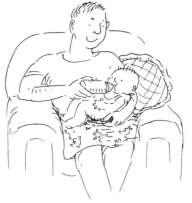

Teething

When your baby is 'teething' (that is, the first teeth start to erupt through the gums), your baby may appear unsettled or unwell.

Children younger than 1 year should never be left in bed with a baby's bottle.

First aid

What to look for
- ➤ excessive drooling
- ➤ red cheeks
- ➤ red, swollen and tender gums
- ➤ child rubbing gums with finger or chewing on another object
- ➤ irritability.

What to do

If your child is unwell, take the child to a doctor to ensure the child does not have a more serious illness. If the doctor says that your child's problems are due to 'teething', make sure that your baby continues to have plenty of fluids.

You can help to relieve some of the discomfort as follows:

1 *Wrap a little ice in a cloth or a handkerchief and place it on your baby's gums. Alternatively, cool a teething ring in the refrigerator (not the freezer) before giving it to your child.*

2 *Give your baby paracetamol according to the directions on the bottle.*

3 *Use a teething gel according to the directions on the packaging.*

145

What the Safety Centre can do for you

If you require further information, or have a question about any of the topics in this book, please write, phone or fax your request to:

Safety Centre
Royal Children's Hospital
Flemington Road
Parkville Vic. 3052
Phone: (03) 9345 5085
Fax: (03) 9345 5086

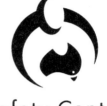

Safety Centre
Royal Children's Hospital

Safety consultants will assist you with your enquiry, or refer you to the most appropriate organisation in your state.

Through this book the Safety Centre aims to improve the health, safety and wellbeing of all Australian children by making parents and carers aware of safety factors and by reducing the number of accidents. The Centre has been working effectively towards this goal since 1979, through education programmes, information and advice, by changing government policy, and designing and advising on safer environments for our children.

The Safety Centre specialises in child, home, school, community and workplace safety. Some of the many services offered include:

- safety-awareness workshops, seminars and short courses
- first-aid and resuscitation courses; including first aid for carers of children, workplace first aid; resuscitation courses and updates
- home-safety shop, which stocks a range of safety products, videos, posters and books (mail order is available)
- telephone advisory service
- national child safety library
- teaching material
- information packages for parents, teachers, students, and carers of children
- model safety kitchen and bathroom
- displays on all aspects of safety, including portable displays
- portable community safety displays
- product and design consultancies.

Index

Index